After Harm

Joseph S. Alper, Catherine Ard, Adrienne Asch, Jon Beckwith, Peter Conrad, and Lisa N. Geller, eds. *The Double-Edged Helix: Social Implications of Genetics in a Diverse Society*

Mark P. Aulisio, Robert M. Arnold, and Stuart J. Youngner, eds. *Ethics Consultation: From Theory to Practice*

Audrey R. Chapman and Mark S. Frankel, eds. *Designing Our Descendants: The Promises and Perils of Genetic Modifications*

Ezekiel J. Emanuel, Robert A. Crouch, John D. Arras, Jonathan D. Moreno, and Christine Grady, eds. *Ethical and Regulatory Aspects of Clinical Research: Readings and Commentary*

Grant R. Gillett. *Bioethics in the Clinic: Hippocratic Reflections*

John D. Lantos. *The Lazarus Case: Life-and-Death Issues in Neonatal Intensive Care*

Carol Levine and Thomas H. Murray, eds. *The Cultures of Caregiving: Conflict and Common Ground among Families, Health Professionals, and Policy Makers*

Thomas May. *Bioethics in a Liberal Society: The Political Framework of Bioethics Decision Making*

Thomas H. Murray, consulting editor in bioethics

After Harm

Medical Error and the
Ethics of Forgiveness

Nancy Berlinger

Deputy Director and Associate for Religious Studies
The Hastings Center
Garrison, New York

The Johns Hopkins University Press
Baltimore and London

The Johns Hopkins University Press
2715 North Charles Street
Baltimore, Maryland 21218-4363
www.press.jhu.edu

Library of Congress Cataloging-in-Publication Data
Berlinger, Nancy.
  After harm : medical error and the ethics of forgiveness / Nancy
Berlinger.
    p. ; cm.
  Includes bibliographical references and index.
  ISBN 0-8018-8167-6 (hardcover : alk. paper)
    1. Medical errors — Moral and ethical aspects. 2. Medical errors —
Psychological aspects. 3. Medical errors — Religious aspects. 4. Physi-
cians — Professional ethics. 5. Physician and patient. 6. Medical ethics.
7. Forgiveness.
    [DNLM: 1. Medical Errors — psychology — Personal Narratives.
2. Ethics — Personal Narratives. 3. Physician-Patient Relations —
Personal Narratives. 4. Religion and Medicine — Personal Narratives.
WB 60 B515a 2005] I. Title.
R729.8.B47 2005
610 — dc22   2004028263

A catalog record for this book is available from the British Library.

To
Andrew Berlinger,
Virginia Ashby Sharpe,
and
Julia Boltin

Contents

Preface

In the years since the release of *To Err Is Human*—the Institute of Medicine's report on the problem of medical error in the United States—made front-page news across the nation in November 1999, it has become almost *de rigueur* for scholars, health care professionals, and journalists to begin their books and articles by invoking the report with its startling statistics on the extent and the cost of the problem.[1] This book is no exception, but my reason for doing so is arguably different from the ritual invocation of the report as shorthand for the "problem of medical error." Rather, I am interested in the implications of the report's title for how physicians, health care administrators, injured patients, and the families of injured patients think, speak, and act in the aftermath of harmful medical mistakes. Clearly, the phrase "to err is human" is intended as a reminder that attempting to eliminate medical error is futile as long as human beings are involved in delivering health care, because making mistakes is part of being human. But it may also remind us of something important about the aftermath of error; notably, the complete aphorism to which the title alludes is "to err is human; to forgive, divine."

When I first heard the title of the IOM report, I naively assumed that the report was going to say something about the nature of forgiveness after medical error—forgiveness being a time-honored, if imperfect and often misunderstood, way of dealing with the aftermath of intentional and unintentional harm between persons and between societies. Finding nothing in the report about this dimension of medical error, and finding nothing in the burgeoning theoretical and empirical literature on forgiveness that addressed the aftermath of unintended harm in the context of health care, I started thinking, talking, and writing about what "forgiveness" might mean in this context. The result is this book.

Forgiveness is a word that signifies "religion" to many people, particularly but not exclusively those who are familiar with Jewish and Christian teachings, practices, and expectations with respect to what ought to happen when one person harms another person. However, these religious teachings, practices, and expectations have permeated secular culture in the West for so long and in so many ways that it is completely natural to talk about error, guilt, shame, confession, apology, repentance, and forgiveness without any reference to religion. Think of any recent confession of wrongdoing by a politician, business leader, or other public figure, which tends to follow this script: Mistakes were made; I am sorry for any pain my actions may have caused, I take full responsibility; I hope those affected by my mistakes will forgive me, find closure, and be healed. Think as well of the post-Watergate lesson reminding public figures that the cover-up is worse than the crime: because a lack of candor breeds suspicion in the minds of others, it is better, ethically and strategically, to tell the truth and accept the consequences than to devote oneself to dissembling, concealment, and lies.

Yet there is more to forgiveness than the clichés trotted out in the aftermath of scandal. It is valid and useful to approach the problem of medical error — in particular, the problem of medical *harm* — from the perspective of how individuals living in this society have long been taught, whether by religion, by other cultural influences, or by their parents, to think about what ought to happen when one person unintentionally harms another person. Most medical harm does not result from the negligence of "bad" doctors. Most physicians feel genuine remorse, even anguish, when they realize that their well-intentioned actions have injured or killed a patient who was under their care, even though they may be in profound conflict about what ought to happen next. They must weigh their obligations toward such patients and their families against their fears about the consequences of fulfilling these obligations.

This book looks at medical harm *from* "error" *to* "forgiveness," with stops along the way at "disclosure," "apology," and "repentance," words that describe the sequence of practices and expectations that may culminate in forgiveness — a voluntary response by the person who has been harmed, in recognition of the sincere words and tangible actions of the responsible person or parties. I am not proposing an ethic of forgiveness in which the harmed person is responsible for bringing about resolution simply by forgiving the person whose actions resulted in harm. Such an ethic would be counterproductive to goals of patient safety as well as neglectful of the concrete needs and responsibilities brought about by harmful mistakes. Rather, I ask — and attempt to answer — the following question: What are the words and actions of individuals and what are the policies and practices of institutions that, if completed in the aftermath of medical harm, may offer injured patients and their families the possibility of forgiving those responsible for the harm?

This book constitutes a religious studies perspective on the aftermath of medical harm in two respects. First, it draws on interdisciplinary work on error, truth telling, apology, repentance, and forgiveness by scholars, both inside and outside the formal discipline of religious studies, who are attentive to the religious roots or dimensions of these themes and to their secular counterparts or expressions. Second, it draws on a particular area of religious studies, Christian social ethics, and the work of a particular Christian theologian, Dietrich Bonhoeffer (1906–1945), whose writings on ethics address many of the questions that are germane to issues of error and forgiveness: What does it mean to tell the truth? Who suffers as the result of harm, and what are our concrete responsibilities toward each of those who suffer? What is the nature of the relationship between a patient and a physician, and between that patient and a health care institution, after that patient has been unintentionally harmed by this physician, in this institution? What is forgiveness, and how can we avoid the temptation of presuming we will be forgiven for our mistakes rather than acting in such a manner as to make it possible for those whom we have harmed to forgive us?

My use of Bonhoeffer's work reflects my own academic background and the ideas that have informed my thinking about the ethics of forgiveness after medical harm, ideas that are readily accessible to readers who may not have a background in religious studies or any knowledge of Christian social ethics. I make no special claims for the intrinsic merit of this or any other religious or theological perspective applied to the problem of medical harm over against secular philosophical perspectives. For example, Bonhoeffer's theory of the "view from below," discussed at the end of chapter 1 and mentioned throughout the book, is not too far from John Rawls's "veil of ignorance," from "standpoint" theories described by Sandra Harding and other feminist philosophers of science, from Michel Foucault's theory of "disqualified knowledges," or from Emmanuel Levinas's ethics of the "Other."[2] Any of these theories has the potential to stimulate fresh and productive thinking about how to improve the care of persons affected by medical mistakes; how to listen for and include different voices and different stories in efforts to resolve individual cases of harm and to make medical education and health care systems more responsive to the needs of injured patients and their families; and how to recognize the Other—the harmed patient, the grieving family, the physician who made the mistake — not as an adversary but in terms of one's responsibilities toward the Other. However, given that attentiveness to religion-derived concepts and practices associated with error and forgiveness may assist in understanding and responding to the needs of persons affected by medical mistakes, it is possible that Bonhoeffer may, by virtue of his vocabulary and commitments, be an especially useful theorist to draw on in addressing this problem, even for readers who do not have any background in religious ethics.

The taxonomy of medical error is vast, colorful, and at times confusing. There are slips, lapses, harmless hits, and near misses; errors of omission and of commission; operator errors, system errors, accidents, complications, and bad outcomes. There are even more elaborate ways to describe and to disguise error: as an "inevitable occasional untoward event," for example. This book does not pretend to offer definitions of medical error that will satisfy all readers and apply to all clinical circumstances; in any case, essential readings on this subject already exist.[3] Rather, my primary focus is on the *experience* of medical *error* (or, in a few cases, suspected error) that results in *injury or other harm* to a patient, or to that patient's family. Although this book makes use of a variety of terms, in most cases, I am writing about medical *mistakes*, those errors defined as "errors of conscious thought" and "misapplied expertise" rather than those defined in terms of poorly designed systems or momentary, unconscious lapses in routines.[4] Mistakes are made by individuals, even if these individuals are working within systems. And they are experienced by individuals: by the individuals who make them, and by the individuals who may be harmed by them. It may, therefore, be helpful to think of this book as an effort to enlarge the accurate but often defensive statement "mistakes happen" to acknowledge the experience of the patient and family to whom harm "happens" as the result of mistakes. The other dimension of medical mistakes that this book addresses, in chapters 3 and 5, in particular, is the harm done to the physician-patient relationship, and to real patients and real physicians, when mistakes are made in the aftermath of an actual or a suspected error, compounding the initial trauma.

Too often, discourse on the problem of medical harm is reduced to a shorthand of "individuals" versus "systems," rather than being discussed in terms of individuals *in* systems, whether that system is a solo practice, a group practice, a community hospital, an academic medical center, or a medical school. This book focuses on the experience of individual clinicians, patients, and family members in the aftermath of medical harm, but it assumes a systems context for these experiences and argues for systems approaches to improving care after medical harm, in particular, with respect to supporting concrete practices such as disclosure, apology, and fair compensation.

Throughout this book, the "clinician" is almost always a physician. To date, most literature and research on the aftermath of harmful mistakes focuses on physicians, who have a professional obligation to disclose mistakes and are accountable for the care of their patients; thus, disclosure is frequently discussed in the literature within the context of the *physician*-patient relationship, not the provider-patient relationship. Although other clinicians — nurses, technicians — may make or be involved in mistakes that injure patients, these clinicians are in a different place in the system's hierarchy and stand in a different relationship to patients. A mistake made by a nurse or a technician would most likely be disclosed by the treating physician or by a hospital administrator. Moreover, nurses and other clinicians, as well as risk managers, clinical ethicists, chaplains, hospital attorneys, and other health care professionals who may be involved in the resolution of medical mistakes, have their own professional cultures, which must be taken into account when proposing changes in the ways individuals within systems respond to needs resulting from medical mistakes. Such are my excuses for limiting the focus of this book to the culture of medicine and its subcultures, with the hope that other health care professionals may find something of use in these pages and that other scholars will take up the challenge of exploring these issues, especially with reference to the culture of nursing.

This book is organized into three parts. Chapters 1 through 3 examine how medical harm is experienced, remembered, and written about by physicians who have made harmful mistakes and by patients and families who have been affected by such mistakes, and propose ways to use these personal narratives in medical education and other settings. These chapters also launch the narrative arc of this book — from error to forgiveness — by offering accounts of what the immediate aftermath of medical error (or suspected error) looks like from the perspectives of the persons most directly affected. We are able to grasp something of the emotional chaos of the immediate aftermath of harmful mistakes when we read a physician's own account of disclosing a fatal error to the patient's family even as the physician could barely comprehend what had just happened; or a surgeon's account of making a mistake while racing against the clock to save a drunk driver's life; or a spouse's account of hearing her husband's surgeon assure her that while her husband's death was "unpleasant" for her, it was *"shattering"* for the surgeon himself; or another spouse's awareness, captured in a deposition transcript, that his wife's death meant he was suddenly the single father of a nine-month-old. We also recognize that the words and actions offered to the patient and family at this time, and thereafter, matter intensely, that there really are right and wrong, appropriate and inappropriate, compassionate and callous, things to say and do. When I discuss these personal narratives with medical students and residents, the story of the surgeon whose idea of comforting a widow was to tell her that he felt worse than she did always gets a strong, almost visceral, reaction. Even if these students and early-career physicians have already learned to be defensive around the issue of medical error and its disclosure ("mistakes happen," "it's all about how you define 'error' "), they recognize that what this surgeon *said* was inexcusable. They don't want to become this kind of physician, and perhaps, having read, discussed, and remembered this story, they won't become him when they do, inevitably, make a mistake that harms a patient.

Chapters 4 through 7 explore each of the sequential steps in the relational process that may culminate in forgiveness after medical harm. The subject of chapter 4 is "disclosure," the very first ethical action that can be undertaken in the aftermath of known or suspected harm, the practice of consistently telling the truth to injured patients and their families. This topic is explored with reference to Bonhoeffer's writings on the morality and meaning of truth telling, one of which he wrote in an effort to understand and defend his own practice of *not* telling the truth in a highly unusual situation. Such a text, and its historical circumstances, may shed light on some of the ways that physicians may justify their own reluctance to disclose mistakes and on their mistrust of efforts to improve disclosure policies and practices within health care institutions.

In discussing "apology," the subject of chapter 5, I draw on the work of legal scholars who have explored the meaning and function of apology in U.S. law and in efforts at conflict resolution. These scholars are sensitive to religious or other traditional definitions of apology and to how these definitions may be at odds with legalistic apology formulas that, while adhering to the letter of the law, may be unsatisfying when they are offered to real human beings.

Chapter 6 explores the nature of "repentance" after harm by examining the always contentious issue of whether, and how, injured patients and their families ought to be compensated for health care needs or lost income resulting from medical mistakes. In examining three different models that aim to deliver fair compensation without litigation, and that integrate compensation into the disclosure of the medical mistake itself, I argue against suggestions that the "magic" of apology ought to be sufficient compensation for patients and families who have suffered tangible hardships resulting from medical injuries and propose that tort reform advocates acknowledge the legitimate needs of injured patients by supporting efforts to deliver fair compensation.

To discuss "forgiveness" in chapter 7, I work from Bonhoeffer's famous condemnation of "cheap grace," forgiveness extended or expected without any acknowledgment of responsibility for another person's suffering or any concrete efforts to alleviate this suffering. In exploring the nature of forgiveness after medical harm, and in arguing for an understanding of forgiveness as the ability to achieve detachment from an incident of harm, I also draw on recent and classic studies of forgiveness, including a study of the professional forgiveness ritual of the Mortality and Morbidity Conference (M&M), whose antecedents in ancient Jewish and Christian forgiveness rituals are obvious, if usually unacknowledged.

The book's concluding section can be approached either as a theory of the ethics of forgiveness after medical harm, or simply as an annotated list of recommendations, practices, observations, and reflections that physicians, medical educators, ethicists, health care administrators, and others may use in thinking about the problem of medical harm and how to improve the care of patients, families, and clinicians affected by this problem. This section is organized in terms of the traditional practices of "confession," inclusive of disclosure, apology, and other methods, both appropriate and inappropriate, of communicating in the aftermath of harm; "repentance," which focuses on actions undertaken to relieve suffering in the aftermath of harm; and "forgiveness," which proposes ways in which individuals and institutions may promote the conditions that may allow injured patients and their families — and clinicians themselves — to detach and move on from incidents of medical harm.

Acknowledgments

This book was inspired by the extraordinary intellectual community that is The Hastings Center, a community of which I am honored to be part, and where I learned to apply my longstanding interest in the religious and cultural dimensions of error and forgiveness to the problem of medical harm. In 2000, the Center launched an interdisciplinary research project entitled "Promoting Patient Safety: An Ethical Basis for Policy Deliberation," which sought to examine the ethical dimensions of the issues that policymakers were beginning to take up in the aftermath of the 1999 Institute of Medicine report on the extent of medical error in the United States. I am deeply grateful to the creator of this project, Virginia Ashby Sharpe, who introduced me to the field of patient safety, and to Raymond Andrews and Lynne Garner of the Patrick and Catherine Weldon Donaghue Medical Research Foundation, who made possible this project and the initial research that led to the writing of this book. I am also profoundly grateful to all of my colleagues at The Hastings Center; in particular, to Thomas Murray, Daniel Callahan, Gregory Kaebnick, and Erik Parens, for their guidance and encouragement, and to Chris McKee and his library staff.

Special thanks are due to Elizabeth Seth and Alissa Lyon, my research assistants; to Ann Mellor, my administrative assistant; to Juniper Lesnik, for tracking down legal references; to Julia Boltin, for sorting out countless citations; to Abby Tannenbaum, for proofreading the manuscript; and to Bette-Jane Crigger, for preparing the index. Nancie Erhard taught me how to write a book proposal, and Joseph Sharples taught me how to write a book.

Mary Anderlik, Carol Bayley, Kris Bryant, Tod Chambers, Virginia Ashby Sharpe, and Dean Weber read portions of the manuscript; Paul Batalden and Jeffrey Rice read the entire manuscript and wrote the reader's guide; Larry Rasmussen, my thesis advisor at Union Theological Seminary, commented on early drafts of the Bonhoeffer material. All of these readers — and every peer reviewer and audience member who ever challenged me to clarify and strengthen my arguments — made my work better. Any mistakes are my own.

The Traveling Fellowship of Union Theological Seminary provided essential funding for research support. Wendy Harris, my editor at the Johns Hopkins University Press, guided this project and this first-time author. I have been deeply fortunate to work with her and her able colleagues, including Nancy Wachter, Linda Forlifer, and Sarah Shepke.

Among the dozens of scholars, patient-safety advocates, and health care professionals it has been my great good fortune to work with on the "Promoting Patient Safety" project and to talk with in the course of researching and writing this book, special thanks are due to Jean Berlin, Charles Bosk, Eric Cassell, Rita Charon, Jonathan Cohen, Donna Conroy, Lyla Correoso, Edward Dauer, Paul Derrickson, Albert Dreisbach, Joseph Fins, Arthur Frank, Sandra Gilbert, Roxanne Goeltz, George Handzo, Curtis Hart, Martha Jacobs, Simon Lee, Carol Liebman, Sandy Spencer, Lee Taft, Leslie Taylor, Dean Weber, and especially Carol Bayley and Albert Wu. All have shaped my thinking and have given me fresh insight into the clinical, legal, social, personal, and spiritual dimensions of error and forgiveness. The listserv of the National Patient Safety Foundation has been another important resource, and I am grateful to its participants and to its moderator, Holly Burt. I would indeed be remiss if I did not thank the Scerbo and Berlinger families for tolerating my habit of introducing medical error into conversations at every family gathering over several years.

Versions or portions of several chapters have previously appeared in the following publications: *Hastings Center Report; Studies in Christian Ethics; Journal of Medical Ethics; Literature and Medicine; Journal of Healthcare Risk Management* (© 2004 American Society for Healthcare Risk Management; reprinted with permission), and *Journal of Pastoral Care & Counseling.* An early version of chapter 7 also appears in the edited volume of essays from the "Promoting Patient Safety" project, *Accountability: Patient Safety and Policy Reform,* edited by V. A. Sharpe (Washington, D.C.: Georgetown University Press, 2004). Permission to use this previously published material is gratefully acknowledged. Versions or portions of several chapters were presented at scholarly and professional gatherings at The Hastings Center, the American Academy of Religion, Narrative: An International Conference, the College of Physicians and Surgeons at Columbia University, the David E. Rogers Health Policy Colloquium at New York Weill-Cornell Medical Center, the Department of Orthopaedic Surgery at New York Medical College, and the Center for Health Care Ethics at St. Louis University.

CHAPTER ONE

Narrative Ethics

Like others who have had traumatic experiences, persons affected by medical mistakes may write and publish their own accounts of these experiences. These stories are rich resources for physicians and other health care professionals, for ethicists and patient-safety advocates seeking to improve the way institutions address the problem of medical harm, for survivors of medical harm, for scholars of health care narratives, and for anyone else seeking to understand what happens *after* a medical mistake injures or kills a patient. What are the medical, financial, emotional, spiritual, interpersonal, legal, professional, and communal ramifications of being harmed by a physician's mistake or of unintentionally harming a patient? How is the same incident perceived and interpreted by each of the persons affected by it? What do patients and families want, need, or expect from physicians after harm? What do physicians want, need, or expect from patients and families after harm? Who is afraid of whom, and why? The answers to these questions can be found in the stories patients, families, and clinicians tell about the mistakes that have touched and, in many cases, permanently altered their lives.

A prominent feature of personal narratives about medical mistakes is the abrupt breaking off, or gradual breakdown, of communications between a physician whose mistake harms a patient and that patient (or family, if the patient has died or become incapacitated). This breaking off or breakdown is usually triggered by or attributed to the physician's or institution's fear that, if injured patients and their families find out "what happened," they will sue. In some stories, it is the unexpected breaking off or breakdown of physician-patient communications that makes a family suspect an error is being covered up. There are other broken aspects to these stories: spiritual brokenness after making mistakes; the fracturing and repairing of patients' trust in caregivers and institutions; the undertow of the hidden curriculum, which teaches medical students and new physicians to break with what they have officially been taught — the professional obligation to tell patients the truth about their health — and to learn, by observing their senior colleagues, how to avoid doing this very thing.

Though physicians have received repeated calls in recent years — from their professional organizations, from patient-safety advocates, from medical ethicists, and from the media — to honor the professional obligation, articulated in the American Medical Association's Code of Ethics since 1981, to disclose mistakes that affect patients' health, empirical studies suggest that most physicians in the United States have not yet been persuaded to do so. Similarly, most U.S. hospitals have not yet been persuaded to embrace and practice the disclosure of harmful mistakes as an institutional obligation.[1] A focus-group survey of physicians' attitudes toward disclosure, conducted in 2002, argues that disclosure may be so far from the norm as to be "uncommon."[2] Although the AMA's Council on Ethical and Judicial Affairs (CEJA) issued a report in 2003 that urged physicians to disclose error, it also acknowledged that, "in today's rough medical liability climate, imparting information about errors seems counterintuitive."[3] As the result of these built-in contradictions — being a physician means you disclose your mistakes, except that being a physician means you don't disclose your mistakes — physicians contemplating disclosure and students contemplating the ethics of being a physician and doing clinical medicine may conclude that their professional obligations and professional norms are irreconcilable. Patients and families affected by harmful medical mistakes, however, may interpret physicians' unwillingness to disclose, apologize for, and acknowledge responsibility for such mistakes as a painful and bewildering lack of compassion, a stance that ultimately is counterproductive as a means of staving off lawsuits.

Narrative ethics — the use of stories, both factual and fictional, to illustrate ethical dilemmas, or to sharpen readers' awareness of voices and circumstances both like and unlike their own — may offer a solution to the problem of what to say and do after medical harm, a problem that has stubbornly failed to yield to appeals to professional ethics. The personal narratives of patients, families, and clinicians (in most cases, physicians), in particular, may, by giving readers insight into the world of the "other" in the aftermath of trauma, offer a way out of the current impasse. Reading and discussing stories written by patients and families may help physicians to understand why disclosure matters so much, and how the failure to disclose and to address other needs resulting from medical harm, is a factor in determining whether to take legal action. Reading and discussing stories written by physicians may help patients and families to understand how a physician experiences the trauma of harming a patient, what physicians fear in the aftermath of harm, and how these fears may affect their subsequent words and actions. As advocacy organizations have begun to call on medical schools and hospitals to involve patients and families in their patient-safety education efforts, such stories may provide a common ground for persons who may not be accustomed to talking *to* one another about mistakes to begin to talk *about* mistakes, and may give them a vocabulary with which to do so. This vocabulary is not derived from the formal language of "obligations," "policies," and "adverse events," but is forged from the words and emotions of the stories' authors. This chapter provides an overview of theories of personal narrative that are relevant to stories of medical error and also to the consideration of the problem of medical error from the perspective of religious studies. The next two chapters will explore, respectively, narratives written by physicians and medical students and narratives written by or from the perspective of injured patients and their families.

The essays collected by philosopher Hilde Lindemann Nelson in *Stories and Their Limits: Narrative Approaches to Bioethics* (1997) provide a useful introduction to the ways in which the overlapping discourses of bioethics, medical humanities, and literary studies approach personal narratives about illness and medicine in general, and for assessing how these critical approaches may (or may not) be useful in reading and interpreting personal narratives about medical error. Within bioethics, the phrase "narrative ethics" usually refers to the argument that a patient's story, voice, and perspective are as important, if not more important, than the clinical account of that patient's treatment as reflected in medical records. Narrative ethicists such as Arthur Kleinman, a medical anthropologist and physician, and Arthur Frank, a sociologist, have described methods for eliciting patients' stories — in Kleinman's famous phrase, their "explanatory model"[4] — of their illnesses, and for reminding physicians that they themselves function as characters in their patients' stories, just as patients function as characters in physicians' stories.[5] Rita Charon, a physician and literature scholar who directs the Narrative Medicine program at Columbia University's medical school, argues that the doing of narrative ethics involves not only eliciting and listening to the patient's story but also recognizing that "duties are incurred in the act of hearing it," in writing it down, and in representing it to other audiences.[6]

Narrative-based approaches to the ethics of the clinical encounter are sometimes reduced, by practitioners and by critics alike, into mere resistance to what is posited as the bastion of "principlism," often represented by the work of Thomas Beauchamp and James Childress, authors of *Principles of Biomedical Ethics*, a book so influential in the teaching and practice of medical ethics that it is itself redacted into shorthand as "Beauchamp and Childress" or "the Georgetown mantra."[7] However, in an essay arguing against the reduction of narrative ethics to mere reaction against principlism, Childress characterizes "narrative(s)" versus "norm(s)" as a "misplaced debate," contending that the influential principles of beneficence, nonmaleficence, autonomy, and justice should not be read as rules that trump any story, given that the principles cannot be honored other than in a narrative context; that is to say, in the context of the physician-patient dialogue.[8] Upholding the principle of autonomy, of respect for the patient's integrity and dignity as a person and a moral agent, always means paying attention to the story a real patient is telling you.[9]

Childress also cautions theorists who are tempted to valorize "narrative" over against "norms"—the story trumps the rules—against what he perceives as an overeagerness to slot patients' stories into "grand" narratives, saying, in effect, your story is not your story, it's the universal quest narrative, or the Christian myth of redemptive suffering, or the worldview of your culture.[10] Religious studies scholar Dena Davis makes a similar point when she cautions clinicians and ethicists against the shortcut of reading the story they know—or think they know, or can look up—about a patient's perceived religion or culture into the real story that this real patient is telling.[11] Applying the principle of autonomy first to "Jewish ethics," for example, or the "Navajo worldview," and thence to your Jewish or Navajo patient, is not at all the same thing as listening to the story of your Jewish or Navajo patient.

The study of narrative is central to medical humanities, a discipline concerned both with the study of literature and other art forms that may take illness and medicine as their subjects, and with the integration of humanistic concerns into the teaching and practice of medicine. Some scholars of medical humanities insist they are literary scholars who are not "doing ethics," whereas Nelson argues that "reflecting on the moral aspects of particular encounters within a powerful social institution" is indeed the stuff of ethics, whether one is comfortable with the word ethics or with making judgments about what ought to happen during these encounters.[12]

In studying narratives of persons writing about their experiences of illness, or narratives that arise from encounters between patients and physicians (or between patients and health care systems in general), scholars of medical humanities frequently draw on literary theory.[13] Literature scholar Anne Hunsaker Hawkins, who has written extensively on the autobiographical genre of pathography — accounts of illness written by the ill person or a family caregiver — has described the uses of this genre.[14] For writers of pathographies, describing their experience is a way of bringing order to the "disordering process" of illness.[15] For caregivers, for survivors of life-threatening illness, and for those who have lost a loved one to illness, reading pathographies is akin to membership in a "vicarious support group," in which reading about the experience of someone who really does seem to know just how you feel may be instructive or comforting.[16] For medical students and clinicians, reading and discussing pathographies serves two functions, according to Hawkins. Pathography helps students "grasp the importance of the assumptions, attitudes, and myths that patients bring to the medical encounter," all the details that may never be elicited during the taking of a patient's history, even by those conscientious clinicians who have read Kleinman on the explanatory model.[17] And incorporating the study of pathography into clinical medicine holds out the promise of "restoring the patient's voice to the medical enterprise."[18] Although Hawkins admits that most pathographies, with the exception of John Donne's *Devotions upon Emergent Occasions* and other narratives written by writers who have experienced serious illness, are not of great literary merit, her theory that reading pathography is good for the moral development of physicians is similar to the theory, advanced by philosopher Martha Nussbaum and by many medical humanities scholars, that reading great literature sharpens the moral sensibilities of the reader and, further, helps the reader to make moral judgments in the world beyond the book.[19]

The discipline known as trauma studies, which pays close attention to the personal narratives of trauma survivors, offers another potential theoretical approach to the study of personal narratives that arise from illness or the clinical encounter. Historian Domenick La Capra, who studies Holocaust narratives and the historiographical challenges of writing about trauma, makes an important distinction between the "event," "experience," "memory," and "representation" of trauma.[20] The traumatic event itself ought not to be conflated with how each of the persons affected by this event experiences it; how each of these persons remembers their experience in the context of other past experiences; and how each of these persons may variously represent their memory, whether in informal conversation, in a published narrative, in a legal deposition, or by other means. Nor can any one person's experience, memory, or representation of the traumatic event be assumed to be the whole factual or moral truth about this event, although one person's experience, memory, or story of trauma may very well function as the "truth" concerning the event for this person and his immediate family and community. La Capra therefore cautions against using personal narratives of trauma to interrogate or discredit witnesses whose stories may not always square with verifiable facts. Writers of trauma narratives have told the story of their experience of an event as they remember it.[21] Further, they have made choices (or have had these choices made for them) concerning the form their narrative will take, and the storytelling conventions associated with this form will further shape the narrative and how it is received.[22]

In applying theories of narrative associated with the doing of "narrative ethics" to personal narratives about medical error, including narratives written by physicians, one must from the outset be aware of a gap in this body of theory. In seeking to restore the patient's voice, whether to the "medical enterprise," as Anne Hunsaker Hawkins sees it, or to the patient herself, as Arthur Frank sees it, narrative ethics does not usually perceive its task as the restoration of the physician's voice.[23] Hawkins is concerned about this gap and does not believe that patients' stories, in which physicians are rarely the heroes, are a reliable source of information about "the inner reality of what it is to be a physician in today's technological medical system."[24] Her influential study of pathography, *Reconstructing Illness*, concludes with this sentence: "Only when we hear *both* the doctor's and the patient's voice will we have a medicine that is truly human."[25]

There is another, larger gap in narrative theory as an approach to the study of personal narratives about medical error and its aftermath. To date, theorists who study personal narratives about illness or the clinical encounter have not yet accounted for those narratives in which the catalyst for the creation of the narrative is not the remembered experience of illness, but rather the remembered experience of a medical mistake that harmed an ill person. These stories, whether they are written by a patient, a family member, or a physician, do not quite fit into the familiar genres that theorists use to describe medical narratives. Unlike pathography, in which the author's experience of her illness and her encounters with the health care system supply plot, narrative drive, and occasions for reflection, a personal narrative about medical error may not be built around the experience of illness, because the very person whose pathography this *would* have been has been killed off, or otherwise displaced from the story, in the early chapters. Also, while authors of pathographies frequently discuss their frustrations with the health care system, personal narratives about medical error are additionally concerned with authors' frustrations (and fears) concerning the *legal* system, a dimension that is especially characteristic of American narratives.

Thinking about illness narratives as occasions for patients to acknowledge that they are more than patients and as tools for creating community among other persons "enacting illness," as well as among the survivors and the temporarily well, as Arthur Frank suggests are the political dimensions of personal narratives, will also take one only so far in developing a theory that encompasses personal narratives about medical error. Although the experience of medical injury is frequently a catalyst for political action on the part of patients and family members, in many cases it is not "illness" that is enacted: persons affected by medical mistakes do not come together in quite the same way as persons living with cancer, HIV/AIDS, or other conditions do. And because the more precise catalyst for political action is usually not merely error or even harmful error, but harmful error that kills or incapacitates a patient, the family member who most frequently "enacts" the role of the person affected by medical error cannot, in most cases, personally reference the lived experience of illness that is so central to illness narratives. Simply put, these enactors may need a different theory.

Relying on trauma studies to provide a theoretical basis for interpreting personal narratives about medical error is problematic as well. Errors that harm patients may indeed be traumatic, whether understood in terms of the impact of the error on the patient's body or in terms of the subsequent impact of the harm to the patient's body on the patient and others. However, theories that are derived from narratives describing the impact of *intentional* harm — abuse, violence, genocide — however useful they may be in helping the reader to understand the phenomenon of trauma, must be used with caution in determining how to respond to the trauma of *unintentional* harm and, in particular, how to address the emotional trauma experienced by the very person whose mistake resulted in harm.

In some respects, personal narratives about medical error are structured more like detective stories, or their nonfiction counterparts, such as investigative journalism, than like any other genre described by scholars of health care narratives. A scene is set: a person goes into the hospital for routine surgery, or arrives at the emergency room with a specific complaint, or is already an inpatient, with a diagnosis and course of treatment. *Something happens.* In many narratives that "something" is the death of the patient. An explanation of what happened is offered, often taking the form of an "official version." There's a problem with this story: gaps in the timetable, missing data, discrepancies between what's recorded in the charts and what the family is told. Suspicions take root. Powerful figures insist that whatever happened was not out of the ordinary, or they refuse to say anything. Family members, friends, and often lawyers scramble to assemble a coherent alternative narrative that will tell them what really happened and who was responsible. There may even be a legal drama, or the prospect of one, as a subplot. There may be an eleventh-hour confession. The truth about what really happened may come out, or it may remain hidden. The personal narrative of medical error, as a hybrid genre, may even incorporate medical records, legal documents, and reconstructed timetables, any of which are stock-in-trade storytelling devices to the writer of detective fiction, as is the narrative thrust provided by the questions, what really happened, why did it happen, and whodunit?

Suggesting that personal narratives of medical error may have parallels in or make use of the genre conventions of detective fiction is not at all to suggest that solving the mystery of a incident of unintentional harm is the same as finding out who committed a crime. Successful detective fiction does not require that a crime be committed for a mystery to be solved or a truth about human behavior revealed.[26] Also, physicians have long been accustomed to approaching and writing about cases as puzzles or mysteries. Recall that the model for the legendary, and fictional, detective Sherlock Holmes was the legendary, and quite real, Professor Joseph Bell of the medical faculty of the University of Edinburgh; that Oliver Sacks describes the telling of "clinical tales" about puzzling cases as part of medicine's deep history; that personal essays in medical journals and general-interest publications alike frequently rely on the conventions of the genre, presenting the physician-writer as detective and the patient's symptoms as the mystery to be solved.[27] However, an important difference exists between clinical tales and personal narratives about medical error. In the clinical tale, the narrative is propelled by the physician-author's reconstruction of her quest to discover the diagnosis or treatment that will improve a patient's health or well-being. Conversely, in a personal narrative about a medical mistake, a patient has almost always been harmed, often irreparably.

This book looks at the moral and practical dilemmas of the aftermath of medical harm through the lens of religious studies, with particular reference to Christian social ethics. As such, before turning this lens on stories written in the aftermath of medical harm, it is fair to ask how paying attention to such stories can be regarded either as religious studies or the narrower category of religious ethics. Stories are an important part of religious and secular rituals associated with the resolution of harm. The Jewish and Christian rituals associated with words such as confession, apology, repentance, atonement, and forgiveness incorporate reciprocal storytelling and listening. After your actions have harmed me, I expect you to tell me what happened, that you regret the harm done to me, and that you acknowledge your responsibility for this harm. For my part, I will listen to your account of what happened and to your apology. You will then listen to me describe how this harm has affected my life, and what I may need to be restored to my former state or to repair my trust in you. I will then listen to you describe how you will effect the reparations or restitution that will heal our damaged relationship.

Our knowledge of these rituals may derive from our own religion and culture, or from the influence of religious norms and practices on what we think of as secular culture: the Mortality and Morbidity Conference, in which physicians tell their peers the story of a mistake or other complication, is recognizable as a ritual that is enacted in a culture that has been greatly influenced by Jewish and Christian norms and practices concerning appropriate responses to harm, even if most of the physicians enacting the ritual of M&M never think of their professional ritual in "religious" terms. Because religious studies scholars seek to identify and understand ritual patterns in the ways individuals relate to that which is beyond the self, a religious studies perspective can be useful in understanding how people who tell stories about medical error perceive themselves in relation to the other characters in their stories, and what they want or expect these characters to do.

When narrative ethics is defined in terms of clinical medicine's moral obligation to pay attention to the voice of the patient, it is very close to the moral standpoint that Dietrich Bonhoeffer calls the "view from below" and describes as the "perspective of those who suffer."[28] Physician David Hilfiker, whose narrative about his own mistakes is discussed in the next chapter, describes something similar to the "view from below" in another article, "From the Victim's Point of

View," in which he argues that learning how to see the medical enterprise from the perspective of the patient is crucial to enabling physicians and other clinicians to "develop an ethical framework in which to work."[29] Bonhoeffer is careful to point out that the "view from below" is not the "partisan possession" of any person or any group who may attempt to stake a claim to being "eternally dissatisfied," or, as our culture might say (and as Hilfiker, a product of our culture, does say) to being "victims." Rather, it is the condition of suffering, whether temporary or permanent, that marks the view from below and also denotes the ethical obligation incumbent on those who are not suffering. Bonhoeffer elsewhere writes that we must recognize the "one who is in concrete distress" as our "neighbor," and further recognize that we have a responsibility to respond to our neighbor's suffering.[30] We cannot merely observe it. We cannot merely feel awful about it. We must act to alleviate it. In David Hilfiker's ethical framework, the "victim" is always the patient, and the patient is always the "victim." In Bonhoeffer's more flexible framework, the suffering of the physician whose mistake harms a patient can also be acknowledged, with the understanding that the "concrete distress" of the patient (and the patient's family) is recognized and attended to first.[31] Bringing this ethical perspective into narrative ethics enlarges the latter's commitments by encouraging its practitioners to make certain that they recognize the voice of the physician as a voice that may also be suppressed, a voice that may also express suffering after harm.

CHAPTER TWO

Physicians' Narratives

Physicians' stories about their own mistakes may take the form of the clinical tale or may be embedded in other familiar genres, such as the memoir or the how-I-became-a-doctor *Bildungsroman* of medical school or residency. In the wake of the Harvard Medical Practice Study,[1] the Institute of Medicine report *To Err Is Human*, and other research that has drawn attention within clinical medicine and among the general public to the problem of medical error in the United States and other developed nations, a hybrid narrative genre has evolved, one that is particularly evident in the leading British medical journals: the error narrative as teachable moment.

The Lancet, for example, now offers a regular feature, the "Uses of Error," consisting of brief essays submitted by clinicians. The moral of many of these essays is summarized by one contributor: "Determination to learn from mistakes, and to make a given mistake only once, is surely a feature of life-long learning."[2] As the name of this feature suggests, these are cautionary tales that "use" mistakes as opportunities to enlighten and instruct one's peers by describing a mistake and what the author learned from it. Many of these essays can also be read as clinical tales built around solving the mystery of a puzzling case, with the solution turning on the resolution of a misdiagnosis or a knowledge gap. Occasionally, a *Lancet* author will address the emotional as well as the didactic dimensions of a mistake. A pathologist writing from the United States describes the aftermath of an early-career mistake that led to a false-positive cancer diagnosis: "I was so mortified that for a week I couldn't even visit the doctors' lounge, fearing everyone was talking about my shameful error."[3] She remembers "an intense desire to go to the patient's room and apologise for my error," which had resulted in unnecessary surgery, and also of her decision that "this was not a good idea in such a litigious society." She concludes the essay by describing how she both atoned for and benefited from this early mistake, the investigation of which resulted in a successful research proposal to study atypical presentations: "I learned a lesson here, and by subsequent research and publications I have tried to educate my peers about my mistake." Another physician based in the United States reminds his peers that their errors cannot be "used" to improve the practice of medicine if they are rationalized as normal outcomes of cases involving very sick or terminally ill patients: "It is very tempting to justify or rationalise an error as a way of not taking responsibility . . . an error that can be rationalised is still a mistake. We must learn from these mistakes to prevent them from happening the next time when the patient is not too sick and the patient is not about to die."[4] This author also describes learning how to deal with an "angry family" as one of the "uses" of error, but also a skill that physicians will never master if they refuse to acknowledge they have made mistakes. For this author, the learning opportunity presented by a mistake is not merely a question of "using" it to improve one's technical abilities, or to refine one's diagnostic skills, or even to avoid making the same mistake twice, but it is integral to the ethics of being a responsible professional who upholds the physician-patient relationship even when it is not at all comfortable to do so.

The other leading British journal, the *BMJ*, also solicits personal essays about readers' own mistakes: "My most informative mistake" is given as a sample title.[5] Yet these essays are quite different from the *Lancet*-style essay, in which the emphasis is on the lesson learned, the unfortunate incident described is often firmly in the past, psychologically and chronologically, and the tone tends to be detached. In the *BMJ* essays, capturing something of the personal and professional turmoil resulting from harming, or having been suspected of harming, a patient is often an important part of the narrative.

In one essay, a U.K.-based general practitioner describes the emotional impact of each stage of the investigation following the hospitalization and death of a patient he had briefly seen in his practice.[6] In dissecting the aftermath of a possible mistake — the title of this essay is "Anatomy of a Complaint" — this author painstakingly describes the effects of fear and anxiety on the body and mind of the physician. Upon learning of the patient's death, he writes that his "emotions were mixed and multiple: shock, sympathy, fear — fear of a mistake, fear of a complaint," and that he was "[w]racked with guilt" as he "mentally tortured" himself, "reliving" his encounter with the patient. When he is notified of the family's complaint, "a crescendo of acute anxiety passed through my body; panic, fear, and shattered confidence engulfed me like a blanket of smoke." His symptoms — "trembling hands, palms sweating, heart thumping, mind racing" — are indeed those of a panic attack, and he later manifests symptoms that he associates with clinical depression: he is "miserable," "unenthusiastic," and "disillusioned." Although the complaint is dismissed, the author assesses this as a "hollow victory," given the "surprisingly dramatic" emotional fallout. He offers advice to his peers, and to himself: "It is essential to share your worries and fears with someone . . . If you are aware of a colleague or friend who is the subject of a complaint it is perhaps your responsibility to take an interest in the problem and provide support and counselling as necessary. Be persistent . . . your initial inquiry may fall on deaf ears."

Another personal narrative published in the *BMJ* also probes the emotional impact of a mistake — in this case, an actual rather than a suspected mistake — on a physician. The author is anonymous, and all identifying details, including the nature of the mistake itself, have been disguised.[7] All we are told is that the author began an emergency procedure on a patient, and, "after half an hour, my patient was dead. At my hands." The author tells us "I was a wreck" after the incident, and that: "The best advice I was given was to write down as much as I could remember as soon as I could. Doing this made me realise how much was just a blur. I remembered impressions, images, emotions much more than a cool sequence of clinical events."

The physician's description of how a fatal error was "remembered" is instructive in and of itself. In terms of understanding what happened, of solving the mystery, it would indeed be ideal if the physician who made the mistake could both remember and describe it as a "cool sequence of clinical events." Yet this narrative suggests that some mistakes — those that are immediately apparent to the physician and that result in immediate harm to the patient — simply cannot be cognitively processed, and therefore cannot be described in a clear, linear way until some time has passed. And when they can be so described, because the physician has convinced himself that the impressions can be resolved into a "cool sequence of clinical events," they may be rationalized as normal events, as occurs in this case.

This observation concerning the disorderliness of a traumatic experience has implications for the disclosure of medical mistakes to patients and families. The author of this narrative describes meeting with the deceased patient's family three times. The author can barely recall the first meeting, immediately after the patient's death, let alone what was said: "I don't know if I was much use to them." Having written down the "impressions, images, emotions" associated with the incident, the author proceeds to get drunk; a colleague, concerned about the possibility of suicide, sits with the author all night. Yet by the next morning, the author has "remembered" the incident as a "normal complication," and meets with the family again, "detailing what happened and why." The third and final meeting with the family takes place after the medical examiner's report suggests the physician may have been at fault: "Armed with the written report I visited the family. Patiently, I explained what went wrong and why. As understanding dawned so did anger. All I wanted to do was cry out, 'It wasn't my fault—I did the best I could.' Instead I listened to the anger directed at me. It was probably justified. It was also the hardest thing I have ever done."

The author charts the emotional landscape of the year after the mistake: the unqualified support of the author's own family; the "mixed" responses of colleagues; the temptations of alcohol; for several months, reliving the mistake through daily thoughts and nightly dreams; collapsing in tears at the realization that " 'getting over it' was not the issue—living with it was"; the disastrous first anniversary, when the author booked multiple procedures ("a mistake") which did not go well ("I was a mess"); the subsequent lessening of anxiety after passing that milestone. The author concludes: "As I write this, the memory still makes my hands shake. The emotions are always there. But . . . I can function and still be an effective doctor. I no longer need the forgiveness I craved at first. I can live with my fallibility . . . But now I truly understand the consequences of failure."

Perhaps the most widely known personal narrative of medical error told from the physician's perspective was written by David Hilfiker, who published an essay in 1984 in the *New England Journal of Medicine* entitled "Facing Our Mistakes."[8] Hilfiker's narrative was, and continues to be, unusual in many respects. It was published well before the recent surge of interest in the problem of medical error and the obligations owed to injured patients and their families. It appeared in a major American medical journal, where personal narratives candidly describing an author's own mistakes, as distinct from scholarly articles about or alluding to mistakes, are still so rare that the word *unique* may apply to this one. And it describes a mistake made by a physician who is established in his career. Hilfiker was 39 years old when his essay was published, six years after the incident it describes at the beginning of the essay. American physicians do publish accounts of errors they made as students or residents, but it is much less common to find more senior physicians writing about errors that cannot be relegated to inexperience.

The story that Hilfiker tells is thus a shocking story, shocking, that a working physician, particularly, an *American* physician, always conscious of living in a litigious society, would publish such an unsparing account of a disastrous mistake — not a "complication," not a suspected mistake — for which he takes full responsibility, using the first person.[9] But because Hilfiker also tells the story of the mistake's aftermath, focusing on the details not only of his own reactions but of his interactions with the patient and family affected by this mistake, it is also a challenging and an oddly hopeful story, in that it compels the reader to notice that the mistake happens to more than one person and to pay attention to how the physician who has made the mistake can and ought to respond to the needs of those most deeply affected by it.

As a general practitioner in a rural practice in the late 1970s, Hilfiker knows his patients well. One patient, Barb Daily, appears to be pregnant, but her urine repeatedly tests negative. Hilfiker considers sending her 110 miles for an ultrasound, then a new technology, but does not; the test is expensive, and he knows that Barb and her husband, Russ, are not well-off. Hilfiker diagnoses a miscarriage and performs a dilation and curettage: during the procedure, he feels "rising panic," and later, a "horrifying awareness" that Barb was, in fact, pregnant and the fetus viable (Hilfiker 1984, 119). Several days after the procedure, when he has received the pathology report, he meets with Barb and Russ, with whom he has been talking all along, telling them "as much as I know, without telling them all that I suspect":

> My consultation with Barb and Russ . . . is one of the hardest things I have ever done. Fortunately, their scientific sophistication allows me to describe in some detail what I have done and what my rationale was. But nothing can obscure the hard reality: I have killed their baby.
>
> Politely, almost meekly, Russ asks whether the ultrasound examination could not have helped us. It almost seems that he is trying to protect my feelings, trying to absolve me of my responsibility. "Yes," I answer, "if I had ordered the ultrasound, we would have known that the baby was alive." (Hilfiker 1984, 119)

Barb and Russ Daily did not file a malpractice suit, even though Hilfiker writes that he is sure they would have won a huge award if they had. Like other physicians writing about their own mistakes, he dissects his fear and his anger concerning what is universally perceived within the profession as an ever-present threat of litigation. "Even the word 'malpractice,'" he writes, "carries the implication that one has done something more than make a natural mistake; it connotes guilt and sinfulness" (Hilfiker 1984, 121). Hilfiker parses other dimensions of guilt, an emotion that he believes most physicians feel after harming a patient, but that he, for one, is reluctant to tell the Dailys, and other patients and families, that he feels. It is, he repeatedly insists, his "burden," and yet he is broken by the weight of this burden on his spirit (Hilfiker 1984, 119, 122). Other physicians echo Hilfiker's uneasiness over whether it is appropriate for physicians to use the disclosure of a harmful mistake as a means of relieving themselves of the burden of making the mistake, and like Hilfiker, may draw on language associated with religion to characterize the dead weight of the mistake and the difficulty in knowing how, or whether, or where, to lay it down. As one physician participating in a focus group on disclosure put it, "[We are] trying to relieve the soul of some burden when we confess our sins or our errors . . . and dumping that onto the patient is not necessarily nice."[10] Yet Hilfiker does not believe that physicians should attempt to deny or repress the powerful psychological dimensions of harmful mistakes, but rather implores his peers to find "psychologically healthy" ways to "address [their] own emotional and spiritual experience" of such mistakes, and indicts the culture of medicine for offering "no place for this spiritual healing" that physicians desperately need, whether or not they acknowledge this need (Hilfiker 1984, 119, 121).

David Hilfiker has a dual vocation as a writer and a physician, and his skill as a writer and his ability to reflect on the meaning of his experience of a harmful mistake, rather than simply to rely on the inherent drama of a mistake as a narrative device, is part of what makes this story so memorable. Two other personal narratives about medical mistakes are notable for having been written by physicians who are also highly accomplished writers. Atul Gawande's essay "When Doctors Make Mistakes" first appeared in the *New Yorker*, then subsequently became a chapter in his memoir of his surgical residency.[11] Danielle Ofri's "M&M" was published in a prominent literary journal before becoming a chapter in her memoir of her medical education and residency at New York's Bellevue Hospital.[12]

There are other similarities between these authors. Both Gawande and Ofri, like David Hilfiker, recognize that mistakes happen to patients and their families, as well as to physicians, and both tell us what they know about the patients and families affected by their mistakes. Both ground their stories about their mistakes within the cultures of their respective specialties (Ofri is an internist) and how these cultures train members to think about mistakes and "complications." And both write at length about the cultural ritual that their specialties rely on to "use" mistakes as teaching tools and to "face" mistakes as an aspect of professional practice: the Mortality and Morbidity (or Morbidity and Mortality) Conference, the "M&M" of Ofri's title. For each author makes a mistake that is presented at M&M, a mistake significant enough to serve as a learning opportunity for their peers and one serious enough to require proof, in the form of public confession, that the author of the mistake takes responsibility for the sin committed.

Several differences between Gawande and Ofri should be considered when reading their stories in tandem. Surgeons and internists have very different jobs and may make very different sorts of errors. They interact with patients and with patients' families differently and may consequently perceive their responsibilities toward patients and families differently. Their respective M&Ms function differently. Although some of these differences may simply reflect practices unique to specific institutions, a recent study comparing how cases involving mistakes were addressed in internal medicine and in surgery M&Ms found that the surgery M&Ms were nearly twice as likely to feature case presentations on errors and other adverse events (72% versus 37%), and that surgeons were far more likely to talk frankly about errors *as* errors.[13] And at the end of the crisis that is narrated in two different idioms in each account — the real-time narration of the resident frantically trying to figure out what is going so badly wrong, and the authorized version of this story as transmitted to the congregation at M&M — Gawande has a living patient, and Ofri does not.

Gawande's story is built around the moral "all doctors make terrible mistakes," a fact acknowledged by the profession, as evidenced by the existence of M&M and by doctors themselves when they are being both honest and candid (Gawande 2002, 55–56). He is careful to distinguish between "good" doctors, who inevitably will make mistakes, and "bad" doctors, who are either incompetent to prevent errors or have ceased to care whether they harm patients.[14] This story, then, is about "good" doctors and about one good doctor in particular, Gawande himself, who is paged to the emergency room one night during his residency to receive a "white female unrestrained driver in a high-speed rollover" (Gawande 2002, 48). The patient, whom Gawande calls "Louise Williams," is "out cold," her breathing "shallow and rapid" (Gawande 2002, 49). We later learn that she was a drunk driver. After an intubation fails, Gawande suspects — or rather, he tells us that he "must have been aware" (Gawande 2002, 50) at some as-yet subconscious level — that the patient's airway is about to shut down and that only an emergency tracheotomy will save Louise Williams's life. He initiates the procedure, which he has never performed on a human patient in an emergency situation (though he had practiced on a goat): "I threw some drapes over her body, leaving the neck exposed. It looked as thick as a tree. I felt for the bony prominence of the thyroid cartilage. But I couldn't feel anything through the layers of fat. I was beset by uncertainty . . . and I hated myself for it. Surgeons never dither, and I was dithering . . . There was no time to wait. Four minutes without oxygen would lead to permanent brain damage, if not death. Finally, I took the scalpel and cut. I just cut. I made a three-inch left-to-right swipe across the middle of the neck . . . I hit a vein . . . I couldn't see anything" (Gawande 2002, 52).

Gawande is unable to open an airway; the surgical attending, Dr. Ball arrives and assesses the situation ("God, what a mess"); the patient goes into cardiac arrest. With seconds to spare inside the four-minute window, the anesthesiologist manages to intubate the patient by using a tube small enough to slip through her swollen vocal cords: "All the people in the room exhaled, as if they, too, had been denied their breath" (Gawande 2002, 54). When Dr. Ball has finally completed the tracheotomy, he speaks with Louise Williams's family: "He told them of the dire condition she was in when she arrived, the difficulties 'we' had in getting access to her airway, the disturbingly long period of time that she had gone without oxygen, and thus his uncertainty about how much brain function she still possessed. They listened without protest; there was nothing for them to do but wait" (Gawande 2002, 55).

Surgical residents responding to emergency trauma cases at 2 a.m. do not have the luxury of getting to know their patients as autonomous persons, and the total time Gawande spent caring for Louise Williams could not have been much more than those crucial four minutes. It's not clear whether Gawande ever saw this patient after she left the emergency room; he tells us only of his "great relief" that she evidently suffered no lasting damage from the botched procedure, that "the episode would heal to a scar" (Gawande 2002, 60–61). Certainly, we cannot hold it against Gawande that Louise Williams is hardly the most sympathetic of injured patients, that she is obese, "with a neck as thick as a tree," that she drove while staggeringly drunk, that she did not wear a seat belt, and that she is unconscious — "out cold" from alcohol as well as the crash — during their entire clinical encounter, which occurred under extraordinarily stressful conditions, in a poorly lit room, in which the person holding the scalpel, who has just made a three-inch "swipe" across the other person's throat, is depending on the memory of a *goat* to help him save this person's life. Our sympathies are likely to lie squarely with the heroic, if hubristic, young surgeon, than with the fat, drunk, irresponsible patient whose brain and life he nearly destroyed because he did not call for help until it was almost too late—and because he made a horizontal, not vertical, incision, which decreased visibility by increasing bleeding.

In telling this story about himself, Atul Gawande's larger project is to illustrate that the Harvard Medical Practice Study, systems theory, and human factors research—the very meat of scholarly and professional responses into why, how, and how often human operators make harmful mistakes—are about "good" doctors like himself and his colleagues, all of whom will make, or barely avoid, disastrous mistakes throughout their careers. A significant portion of his essay is therefore dedicated to exploring how various medical specialties, including his own, grapple with the "paradox of error," in which techniques to avoid mistakes can be perfected, but the human beings who use these techniques cannot (Gawande 2002, 72).

Danielle Ofri's project is different. Her essay "M&M" is prefaced with a quotation from Wordsworth: "But from these bitter truths I must return / To my own history."[15] Ofri's focus never strays from her "own history" of the incident that led to her presentation at M&M. This is her own history in two senses. We see everything, moment by moment, through her eyes; there are no dispassionate detours into systems theory, as in Gawande's essay. And we read her own history, her secret history, of the incident as an untamed gloss on the terse text of her M&M presentation. It is a brilliant display of storytelling technique, the "cool sequence of clinical events" demanded by the narrative and professional conventions of M&M ceding to an italicized inner monologue, in which Ofri describes not only her own "impressions, images, emotions" over the harrowing night she tried and failed to save Raphael Herlan, but also much about Mr. Herlan himself.

Ofri meets Mr. Herlan after he was admitted to the hospital; she was the medical consult on duty that weekend, nearing the end of her residency in internal medicine. Mr. Herlan had an unusual medical history. After he had attempted to kill himself by swallowing lye, surgeons rebuilt his destroyed esophagus by using a portion of his colon. This reconstructed section occasionally needed to be reopened with balloon dilatation, and he had undergone this procedure shortly before Ofri went on duty. She meets him on a Saturday evening, after being informed by the intern on duty that the patient's blood pressure was low. She is "impressed" to see that Mr. Herlan has finished the notoriously difficult Saturday *New York Times* crossword puzzle (Ofri 2003, 191). Despite his protestations — *"Really Doc . . . I feel okay"* — she is concerned by his elevated lactate, as the body produces lactate only when starved of oxygen (Ofri 2003, 191). She transfers Mr. Herlan to the intensive care unit after checking with the attending in charge, who is at home: *"No attending . . . ever wants to get sued — he said okay"* (Ofri 2003, 191). The text of the M&M presentation states merely that "the patient was anxious"; Ofri's "own history" is more revealing:

> *Mr. Herlan pestered me as we wheeled his stretcher down the hall . . . He twisted his head on the pillow so that he could see me better. "I'm not really that sick, am I?"*
>
> *Why do patients always ask these questions? How can you answer honestly without scaring them?*
>
> *Mr. Herlan reached for my hand. "I'm kind of nervous, doctor . . . Do you think you could call my friend John at home? Don't make it sound bad, but I'd like him to come to the hospital. Would you mind?" I nodded as we entered the ICU.* (Ofri 2003, 192)

As the M&M text indicates, at this point "technical difficulties" (Ofri 2003, 193) begin. Ofri is unable to insert a huge Swan-Ganz catheter in Mr. Herlan's jugular vein — *"Just go in, damn it! I pushed and twisted and goaded and prayed"* — and so must do without internal blood pressure readings as she tries to solve the mystery of why his blood pressure is continuing to drop (Ofri 2003, 193). She suspects an esophageal rupture or a tiny perforation from the balloon dilatation procedure has triggered an infection, but fears Mr. Herlan is too unstable to be moved for an X-ray that could confirm this possibility. Ofri orders one drug to elevate blood pressure, then another, then another, plus multiple antibiotics and other medications. Mr. Herlan's anxiety increases with each new procedure:

> *"I'm okay, really, I am . . . I'm going to be okay, right?*
>
> *What's going on, Doc? This is making me really nervous . . . I'm feeling really scared, Doc. Really scared.*
>
> *"Please, Doc. You gotta help me." Mr. Herlan grabbed my hand forcefully and pulled himself up. There was a wild look in his eyes. "Please, I'm not going to make it otherwise. I'm really, really scared. Hospitals always make me scared."* (Ofri 2003, 194-5).

Mr. Herlan becomes so agitated that he is unable to breathe. Ofri orders intubation and increasingly heavy sedation: *I tried to explain why we had to do this, but he clawed desperately at us. I held him down and rubbed his chest . . . Tears were running into his oxygen mask . . . Reluctantly, I turned to the anesthesiologist. "Put him out"* (Ofri 2003, 196).

The crises cascade. Mr. Herlan's lungs fill with fluid, he appears to be having a heart attack, and he continues to fight the breathing tube. Ofri orders a paralyzing sedative and still more drugs to elevate his blood pressure. Mr. Herlan's partner, John, arrives: *"How to say that the patient is crashing and the doctors don't have a clue"* (Ofri 2003, 199). By 2 a.m., eight hours after she first began to treat Mr. Herlan, Ofri has persuaded the covering attending to come to the hospital. He is unable to diagnose the problem that has triggered the near-complete shutdown of Mr. Herlan's system and directs Ofri simply to keep the patient comfortable. She breaks the news to John, who asks to spend the next few hours at the bedside: *"I accompanied John to the ICU, but when I saw Mr. Herlan, I had John wait at the door"* (Ofri 2003, 201). Ofri and the nurse remove some of the IVs and monitors and conceal others under blankets and pillowcases. They clean Mr. Herlan, change his gown, and comb his hair. *"Then, I called John in"* (Ofri 2003, 201).

When Ofri returns to the hospital on Monday morning, having spent 30 hours on duty, she learns from the chief resident that Mr. Herlan is dead and that the catalyst for the crisis was indeed an esophageal rupture:

> *"Oh, Mr. Herlan? He had free air in his heart. That's why he went into cardiogenic shock and died . . . It's in the X-ray report. Didn't you read it?"*
>
> *. . . Could I have missed that? . . . I had examined every single X-ray myself.*
>
> *But I hadn't, I realized with rising nausea, read the written X-ray reports.*
>
> *Usually, the radiologists call immediately if they see an "emergency" problem. As the clinician, however, it was still my responsibility to read the X-ray reports in addition to examining the actual X-rays. It wasn't the radiologist's fault, it was mine. I killed Mr. Herlan.* (Ofri 2003, 204)

Ofri ends her M&M presentation by reading from the X-ray report and acknowledging that she had failed to read the report while treating the patient. Then, in an extraordinary plot twist, the radiologist, who is also in the room, confesses two mistakes of her own. She had failed to call the physicians treating Mr. Herlan as soon as she spotted the free air in the X-ray. And she had misread the X-ray. What had initially looked like free air was, as Ofri had concluded, merely a shadow from the section of colon used to repair Mr. Herlan's esophagus after his suicide attempt. Therefore, although Ofri made a technical error in failing to read the X-ray report, the report itself was incorrect, and treating Mr.

Herlan for a nonexistent rupture would not have saved his life. The head of the Internal Medicine department sums up the case by concluding that a microperforation in Mr. Herlan's repaired esophagus had introduced intestinal bacteria into his bloodstream, leading to a catastrophic, though undetectable, infection. Thus, in the eyes of this most senior physician: "Mr. Herlan died of his own hand. It took three years for his suicide attempt to be completed, but it finally killed him" (Ofri 2003, 207).

Ofri describes herself as seething with anger toward the staff physicians who had "abandoned" her and her patient: "I was crashing on that night also. Couldn't they have helped me?" (Ofri 2003, 205, 206). But, mindful that she had to work with these same physicians, she does not express her outrage, although she feels "an overwhelming urge to disembowel someone with my own bare hands" (Ofri 2003, 207).

Although the Mortality and Morbidity Conference itself is one of the locations in which this story is enacted, Danielle Ofri says little about the effectiveness of M&M as a vehicle for confronting and learning from mistakes, other than to refer to herself as that week's designated "victim" (Ofri 2003, 188), and to comment sarcastically on how residents like herself are expected to embrace the experience of being the "victim": "when something goes wrong, who gets tossed into the fire at M&M? After all, this is an academic institution, and we're here to learn!" (Ofri 2003, 189). Atul Gawande, by contrast, believes in M&M as the "one place . . . where doctors can talk candidly about their mistakes, if not with patients, then at least with one another," and asserts that, of all medical specialties, surgeons are most inclined to "take the M&M seriously" (Gawande 2002, 57). His description and experience of M&M could not be more different from Ofri's. Whereas Ofri presents to an audience that includes representatives of many different areas of the hospital, including legal affairs, Gawande, in describing the audience for surgery M&M, mentions only the surgeons and students on surgical rotation. Ofri presents in a fluorescent-lit conference room; Gawande describes an entirely more ennobling, if potentially more intimidating, environment. The surgeons meet in a "steep, plush amphitheater lined with oil portraits of the great doctors whose achievements we're meant to live up to. All surgeons are expected to attend . . . The chairman is a leonine presence" on the podium (Gawande 2002, 58). The most significant difference, however, is that at Gawande's hospital, the chief residents present all cases, and, according to the norms of the culture of surgeons, the attending in charge of the case must take responsibility for all mistakes. At Ofri's hospital, she must present the case herself, and there is no expectation that an attending will take responsibility for the outcome of Mr. Herlan's case: rather, "it's always the resident who gets flayed for the screwups" (Ofri 2003, 189). Gawande can therefore observe the performance of M&M—albeit from the last row, embarrassed and ashamed—in a way that Ofri cannot. He is in the audience; she is onstage. From his perspective, the show, as a performance designed to instruct, and, by the fact that it never closes, to bear witness to the inevitability of mistakes, is a success.

Chapter 7 will look more closely at M&M as a cultural ritual with deep, if often unacknowledged, roots in religious practices and expectations concerning appropriate responses to human error. In the present discussion of the stories that persons affected by mistakes create and tell, the way that a story is constructed and presented at M&M is of particular interest. Atul Gawande writes that these presentations are "bloodless and compact," and that a "successful M&M presentation inevitably involves a certain elision of detail and a lot of passive verbs" (Gawande 2002, 59). Thus, he comments on the chief resident's M&M presentation of Gawande's own mistake: "No one screws up a cricothyroidotomy. Instead, 'a cricothyroidotomy was attempted without success.' The message, however, was not lost on anyone" (Gawande 2002, 59). The use of technical language and the passive voice to disclose mistakes to patients and family members, as distinct from their use within the closed professional ritual of M&M, where everyone speaks and understands this language, is an ethically charged issue. Medical jargon can be both unfamiliar and intimidating, and even when a physician does, technically, disclose a harmful mistake, injured patients and their families may have no idea what they are being told and no confidence in their ability to ask questions. Researchers who conducted the aforementioned focus-group study of physicians' attitudes toward disclosure wrote that the physicians in the study "spoke of 'choosing their words carefully'" when discussing errors with patients and that this phrase in most cases described practices that would tend to conceal rather than disclose that the physician was talking about a mistake.[16] These physicians claimed that patients would ask questions if they wanted more information about an "adverse event"; however, patients in the same study said that they wanted "basic information [to] be provided to them rather than having to ask their physician numerous questions."[17] David Hilfiker questions whether even the "emotionally mature physician" who wants to honor the obligation to disclose a harmful mistake can explain certain mistakes in ways that patients and families can understand, and further, whether this physician is permitted by the culture of medicine to offer a "real confession," saying plainly,

" 'This is the mistake I made; I'm sorry' " (Hilfiker 1984, 121). Writing 20 years ago, Hilfiker concluded that such a statement "doesn't fit into the physician-patient relationship" as then conceptualized (and controlled) by the culture of medicine. As will be discussed in chapters 5 and 6, this norm may be changing, due in part to demands by patients and families to hear such "confessions," and in part to the efforts of some health care institutions to support physicians in the practices of truth telling and apology.

In the rigid hierarchy of clinical medicine, medical students learn by observing interns, who learn by observing residents, who learn by observing attendings. This hidden curriculum transmits powerful messages about what to say and do — and what never to say and do — on the subject of mistakes. Reading physicians who write about their indoctrination into the culture of medicine, we learn, as all physicians learn, very early in their careers, the euphemisms for error: a mistake is a "significantly avoidable accident,"[18] or an "inevitable occasional untoward event,"[19] or an "unfortunate complication of [a] usually benign procedure."[20] We learn how being tapped by a senior surgeon to be the "keeper of secrets" following a postsurgical mistake that had killed a cardiac patient made one third-year medical student, the lowest of the low, "feel special — an entrusted colleague, a real doctor."[21] We learn that fears of litigation, of becoming a "medico-legal sitting duck," shape different narratives, including the patient's chart and any other documents that could be seen by patients or their lawyers.[22] We learn that the hidden curriculum teaches students and residents how to compose and contribute to successful narratives about mistakes, when success is measured in terms of personal and institutional protection from litigation or in terms of transmitting tribal norms. What we do *not* learn from these stories is whether the hidden curriculum is capable of teaching early-career physicians how to tell injured patients, and their families, what happened, why it happened, and who was responsible, with clarity, candor, and compassion. Nor do we learn whether the hidden curriculum can show these physicians how to acknowledge and deal with their own emotions in the aftermath of harm — in particular, with the sense of shame that Atul Gawande captures in the phrase, "I was what was wrong" (Gawande 2002, 61).

Some medical educators are experimenting with narrative-based approaches to help practicing physicians come to terms with errors they have made. In one model, physicians write out the story of a mistake, omitting their own names. The stories are then collected by the facilitator and distributed randomly among group members, who take turns reading each other's stories aloud.[23] In another model, physicians also write out the story of a mistake, but in the form of a letter to the patient or family affected by it. They then read their own letters aloud.[24] Although both models encourage physicians to acknowledge their mistakes, presumably without taking refuge in the passive voice or other conventions of the "successful" if "bloodless" M&M version of the story, the second model both compels physicians to take responsibility for their mistakes, by reading their own stories, and to recognize that the mistake also happened to the patient and family, by writing the story as a letter. It is possible to imagine pushing these models even further, by integrating them with the "Parallel Chart" technique developed by Rita Charon,[25] in which third-year medical students who are completing their clinical rotations write about the patients they are caring for, learning, in the process, how to recognize and respond to these patients as persons, rather than as " 'the disease in the body in the bed.' "[26] It is not too much of a stretch to envision a group of medical students or physicians writing the story of a mistake twice, first from their own perspective, and then from the perspective of "those who suffer," the perspective of the injured patient and the patient's family.

However, if it is too difficult, whether for students, physicians, or educators, to envision creating parallel narratives of medical harm — and, in so doing, to acknowledge that their own story of mistake is never the only story of the mistake — reading stories that fully acknowledge the impact of medical harm on physicians and on patients may help clinicians to reconcile their own fallibility ("mistakes happen") with the painful reality that mistakes "happen" to patients as well as to their doctors. When the trauma experienced by injured patients and their families is unacknowledged or actively suppressed by individual physicians, by the culture of medicine, or by health care systems, the person most traumatized by a medical mistake becomes the person who made the mistake. It is abundantly clear from the stories discussed in this chapter that physicians are affected, even traumatized, by mistakes that harm patients. But in too many institutions, a patient, once harmed, is no longer thought of or treated as a person with medical problems, in need of care and compassion, or as a person who has suffered a further trauma that may have tangible medical and financial repercussions. Instead, this patient and this patient's family are now thought of and treated as legal problems for the institution. Physicians, nurses, chaplains, and others whose vocation is the care of the sick may be instructed, or may learn through the hidden curriculum and through institutional culture, that they must *never* speak with injured patients and their families. Even hospitals that do formally disclose harmful errors to patients and families may balk at allowing individual physicians to apologize to patients or to acknowledge any personal responsibility for their own mistakes. As will be discussed in the following chapters, many of these taboos are rooted in fears and myths concerning liability, but they also persist because it is painful to acknowledge the injured patient's experience, to listen to the injured patient's voice, and to respond to the injured patient's needs.

Proponents of alternatives to litigation after medical harm speak of "dealing the patient back in,"[27] making the patient a participant in seeking a just resolution to the harm, rather than assuming that the only standpoint an injured patient can have, with respect to a health care provider, is that of angry (and greedy) litigant. Medical educators, as well as ethics educators and others responsible for improving the way health care professionals respond to medical harm, can also deal the patient back in, by using stories about medical harm to reintroduce the patient's voice and the patient's experience into conversations and training around the troublesome issue of disclosure, and in so doing, repositioning disclosure itself as a conversation that is properly understood as part of the physician-patient relationship, rather than as a professional obligation that all too often is sabotaged by the hidden curriculum. David Hilfiker writes that he spoke to Barb Daily's husband immediately after the disastrous procedure, and kept talking to Barb and Russ all week while waiting for the pathology report that confirmed his immediate suspicions. His formal disclosure to the Dailys was embedded in this ongoing dialogue: he had never stopped being in a relationship with them, and he had never stopped telling them the truth ("as much as I know") and being mindful of their crushing loss. He maintains this relationship, and his attentiveness to the Dailys' rights, needs, and suffering, even as he is conscious that his own suffering will not be assuaged through this relationship: his wounded spirit is not the Dailys' problem to solve. Danielle Ofri tells a story that residents, in particular, can identify with: a physician who is building and honoring a compassionate truth-telling relationship with Mr. Herlan and his partner, even as she is desperately trying, and failing, to save Mr. Herlan's life, and agonizing over whether she is making mistakes that are contributing to the crisis. Atul Gawande tells a story that forces the reader to reassess his or her own definition of the physician-patient relationship and what this relationship can reasonably encompass, in light of Gawande's total interaction with Louise Williams: four minutes with an unconscious patient in the middle of the night.

A clear moral role exists for the personal narrative of medical harm as a tool for encouraging medical students and physicians to be ever mindful of the continuing impact of their mistakes on many lives, including, but not limited to, their own lives, and for helping them to perceive and acknowledge their concrete obligations to patients and families after harmful mistakes. But stories written by physicians, about physicians, in most cases for physicians, can tell only one side of the story of a mistake. The personal narratives of injured patients and their families are also crucial tools for dealing the patient back in. These stories are the subject of the next chapter.

CHAPTER THREE

Patients' and Families' Narratives

Personal narratives about medical error that describe the experience of injured patients and their families may be published as essays in peer-reviewed health policy journals or in newsletters for patient-safety advocates. They may take the form of memorial Web sites. They may be shaped into advertisements by activists. They may be read during legislative hearings and become part of the congressional record. They may be as brief as a caption in a photo essay. They may be book-length memoirs. One of these narratives incorporates nearly one thousand pages of documents and was still growing nearly a decade after the patient's death.

Patients' stories about the aftermath of medical harm are often written by family members for a reason that quickly becomes obvious to the reader: the injured patient is dead or is otherwise unable to remember and write her own story. Mindful of Domenick La Capra's taxonomy of trauma, described in chapter 1, which demarcates the "experience," "memory," and "representation" of a traumatic "event" from the event itself, it is worth thinking about the extent to which an "experience" and a "memory" of medical harm happen to a patient's family (and, indeed, to that patient's physician), particularly if the patient does not consciously experience the harm or retain any memory of it — or never forms a memory of it, because the harm was fatal.

In her memoir *Wrongful Death*, literature scholar and poet Sandra Gilbert describes the precise moment when she and her family began to experience medical harm, the moment that they learned that Gilbert's husband, Elliot, was dead following surgery for prostate cancer:

> The surgeon, an Irishman, becomes oddly hearty.
>
> "We've had a problem, luv, a *big* problem," he begins briskly, as he steers me out of the lobby and down a hospital hall I didn't know existed.
>
> I managed to say "What — what — ?"
>
> "Dad's had a heart attack," he replies, shaking his head with what seems to be strange ruefulness.
>
> "But what, but what are you — ?" I begin.
>
> In the background, from the pastel depths of the empty late-night hospital hallway, I hear the screams of my daughters, who are talking separately to the white-coated resident.
>
> . . . I begin to cross myself compulsively. "Are you trying to tell me, Doctor," I whisper, "that my husband is *dead?*"
>
> In the lobby, one of my daughters has flung her shoulder bag across the floor . . . She and her sister and her sister's roommate are screaming and screaming.[1]

The family is brought to the bedside and shown Elliot's body. "I know, I know, for you this is unpleasant, awful," the surgeon tells them, "but believe me for me it's *shattering*" (Gilbert 1997, 39, 72, 337). Recalling this remark later, Gilbert asks herself, "What did he mean? Did he really mean that the doctor is even more pained than the 'bereaved'?" (Gilbert 1997, 72). In the following weeks, Gilbert receives several unsolicited phone calls from the surgeon. During the first call, he tells her the autopsy has taken place, and that "the operation was successful" and "we made the right decision" (Gilbert 1997, 78). During the second call, he reports that he's received the pathologist's report, which confirms that "the surgery was a complete success" (Gilbert 1997, 111). Five times during this brief conversation, the surgeon asserts that neither he nor his surgical resident knew why Elliot Gilbert died hours after successful surgery.

With the help of a physician friend, who reviewed her husband's medical records and noticed some inconsistencies, and, eventually, through a lawsuit, Gilbert learned that her husband died of internal bleeding in the recovery room despite being given twelve units of blood, and that a hematocrit, which might have revealed the bleeding, was delayed for several hours. Neither the hospital nor the surgeon ever told her that an operating room error precipitated the crisis. As an accomplished literary stylist, Gilbert is particularly good at capturing the sleuthing involved as family, friends, and, eventually, attorneys attempted to solve the mystery of her husband's death — poring over the autopsy report and, later, the deposition transcripts; noting unusual language and wondering if it suggested a "cover-up" (Gilbert 1997, 140); piecing together a time line of Elliot's last hours; and, as the denouement, identifying the terrifying gap in the time line, the hours that the hematocrit went missing. But these conventions of the detective-fiction genre are interwoven with inner monologues and descriptions of heart-rending grief. Here is Gilbert, reflecting on the meaning of the missing blood test: "*baby, if they let you lie there for three-and-a-half hours with a hematocrit of seventeen, they killed you, baby*" (Gilbert 1997, 278).

Carol Levine, herself a prominent bioethicist, describes an incident of medical harm and the events that led up to her decision to file a malpractice suit, in her essay, "Life But No Limb: The Aftermath of Medical Error."[2] Like Sandra Gilbert, she tells a story about a mistake that harmed her husband, but, as Levine tells us, "It is my story because the person to whom direct harm was done is unable to give his own account" (Levine 2002, 237). Levine's husband was gravely injured in a car accident, of which he has no memory. During his hospitalization, two catheters were placed in his right hand, blocking circulation; as the result of this mistake, his right hand and forearm had to be amputated. Levine recalls how she was told about the error:

> . . . the neurosurgeon met me in the hall. He seemed very angry. "There was a mistake," he said. "The catheter used to measure arterial gases became clogged, and a new catheter was placed on the same hand instead of the other hand. You never put two sticks in one hand. When that catheter became clogged, circulation was blocked through his hand."
>
> He then said, "It wasn't noticed for twenty-four hours," the passive voice subtly deflecting responsibility from a human agent. . . . "They'll fix it. It's not life-threatening." I asked, "But it is hand-threatening, isn't it?" He only shrugged and walked away. (Levine 2002, 238)

Levine's attentiveness to the surgeon's use of the passive voice and refusal to state explicitly that the mistake was indeed "hand-threatening" reminds the reader of Atul Gawande's similarly fine-tuned observation that, among surgeons, the "successful" presentation of a bad outcome "inevitably involves . . . a lot of passive verbs."[3]

Levine writes that she filed a lawsuit in part because a settlement would allow her to care for her husband, who was greatly impaired as the result of the original accident as well as the loss of his hand, at home. But she also tells of feeling "abandoned and aggrieved" after being "stonewalled" for two years by physicians, lawyers, and administrators: "Doctors and risk managers underestimate both the importance that families place on knowing what happened to loved ones and the frustration they feel when stonewalled. If there were more openness, including apologies, some lawsuits might be forestalled and others settled quickly, without so much emotional toll on families and physicians. Our lawyers have reconstructed a fairly good but still incomplete picture of what happened to my husband; to this day we do not know the details" (Levine 2002, 241).

Contrary to myth, only a tiny percentage of injured patients ever sue their doctors. The Harvard Medical Practice Study, which examined the records of more than 30,000 patients, found that less than two percent of patients who had been injured filed malpractice claims.[4] The study's authors concluded that "medical-malpractice litigation infrequently compensates patients injured by medical negligence."[5] However, as will be discussed in chapter 6, because U.S. hospitals rarely offer compensation to injured patients without legal action first being initiated, the tort system, as Carol Levine points out, is often the only option available to those patients and families who may need compensation because of the continuing medical or financial ramifications of the original mistake (Levine 2002, 241). In many American narratives about the aftermath of medical harm, the question of whether to sue is simply part of the story, forced on the narrator and the narrative by the perceived lack of alternatives to litigation, whether as a means of compensation or as a means of finding out what really happened. But this aspect of the story cannot, and should not, be reduced to or conflated with the myth that "everybody sues." Because "everybody" does not sue.

The stories told by Sandra Gilbert and Carol Levine, though different as to length, form, and, to some extent, readership and purpose, are similar in several respects. In addition to the shared perspective (wife of injured patient), both stories describe cases in which there was clear evidence of error and in which litigation followed on the hospital's failure to fully explain what happened, and, in Levine's story, to address her husband's long-term need for care. In other stories written by family members, it is the treatment of the family after a patient's death that the family views as a mistake, and even as suspicious, although whether a medical error contributed to the patient's death cannot be confirmed.

Michael Rowe, a sociologist and clinical professor at Yale School of Medicine, describes such a scenario in an essay about his teenaged son Jesse's death after two failed liver transplants.[6] Rowe was deeply distressed by what he perceived as a "lack of empathy" on the part of Jesse's doctors following the death. Their failure to contact the family, after weeks of constant contact during Jesse's hospitalization, began to suggest guilty knowledge, as "trust died and mistrust took its place" (Rowe 2002, 235). Rowe recalls his speculations: "What if Dr. Dorand and the others didn't want to talk to us because they had made mistakes that had cost Jesse his life? What if the perforation that occurred during Jesse's first liver transplant was not a 'surgical accident,' as Dr. Dorand had described it, but a surgical error?" (Rowe 2002, 235).

Rowe does look into filing a lawsuit, but his attorney declines to take the case after a liver specialist concludes that negligence, though a possibility, would be hard to prove. Like Carol Levine, he sorts through his feelings about what survivors of known or suspected medical error are trying to say when they file lawsuits, or think about filing them: "many of those who sue doctors, as well as many of those who do not, have no place else to hand their grief when that grief — and seemingly their loved one's life — is being ignored, even declared, in the space left by silence, a thing of no value" (Rowe 2002, 236). And like Levine, he is attentive to the "emotional toll" that medical harm exacts on all parties, concluding his story by suggesting that "both doctors and family members might benefit from words and actions that bridge the silence that death leaves behind" (Rowe 2002, 236).

Roxanne Goeltz's story of her brother Mike's death was initially published in the newsletter of the National Patient Safety Foundation and was subsequently read into the record of a U.S. Senate hearing on patient safety.[7] Mike had gone to the emergency room of the hospital in his small midwestern town one afternoon, suffering from severe stomach pain. After several hours in the emergency room, he was admitted and given a self-administered morphine drip. Early the next morning, his parents, who lived in the same town and had accompanied him to the hospital, received a call from the hospital, "telling them Mike was not doing so well."[8] When they arrived, rigor mortis had already set in, suggesting that Mike had died some hours prior to the call. When Mike's parents saw his body, the arm with the intravenous tube was dangling down the side of the bed. Distressed by this sight, his father "tried to put Mike's arm under the sheet but was unable to bend it."[9] No one from the hospital accompanied Mike's parents to the bedside; instead, Goeltz writes, "my parents were allowed to go to the body of their dead son with no one there to support them."[10] The contrast with Danielle Ofri's description of preparing her living but nonresponsive patient, Mr. Herlan, to be seen by his partner, John, could not be more stark. Ofri had "accompanied John to the ICU," but then glances into Mr. Herlan's room and sees what Mr. Herlan looks like after hours of desperate interventions: tubes and machines connected to every part of his body, a sweat-drenched gown and disheveled hair, syringes, bandages, and other detritus.[11] She sees Mr. Herlan as John would have seen him, had she not accompanied him to the room; then, recognizing how profoundly distressing this sight would be to a patient's partner, she acts quickly to prepare the patient and the room so that John can bear to enter it and sit at the bedside for the rest of the night.

Apart from being told that their son died of "blood around the heart" and that the emergency room had been busy that day, Mike's parents were never given a clear explanation of the events that led to Mike's death, or whether the family history of aneurysm that Mike's mother had given to a nurse was ever taken into consideration.[12] Goeltz describes the implications of the hospital's handling of Mike's death, on her parents and on their close-knit community, in which everyone knew — and didn't know — what had happened to their son and friend at the local hospital:

> A community in shock. Mike has so many friends, they want answers too, they are angry. Those that could give some answers hide behind the hospital doors. The hospital administrator, who attends church with my parents, offers no condolences. Is this the kind of person who is in charge of caring for their community's health? We are able to forgive mistakes but not indifference, not denial and hiding. So many people calling and stopping in to see my parents, trying to understand, offering condolences and support. Mike is gone and we cannot understand what happened, the hospital has no explanation, no apology, no condolences, and no help to try and deal with the loss. Why are the family members ignored, shunned and treated by the responsible facility as if they are at fault?[13]

As in so many American stories about medical mistakes, the lawsuit enters into the narrative of Roxanne Goeltz and her family as a tool of detection, a way of finding out what really happened. Like Michael Rowe and his family, Goeltz and her family interpret the hospital's silence as possible evidence of guilty knowledge. "Our initial reaction" to this silence, Goeltz writes, "was to get a lawyer, so we could get some answers."[14] And as in Rowe's story, faith in the lawsuit as a plot-solving device is extinguished when Goeltz's family is told, by an "out of town lawyer" the family consulted after finding that no local lawyer "would touch" the case, that there was no conclusive evidence of negligence, and also that any settlement would be so small as to be "not worth the work" that the lawyer would need to do.[15]

Roxanne Goeltz is an air traffic controller. In the weeks after her brother's death in September 1999, two months before the Institute of Medicine report *To Err Is Human* became page-one news, she did an Internet search on "medical error," a phrase she had never heard before, and came up with exactly one hit, the National Patient Safety Foundation Web site.[16] She attended a regional conference on patient safety, where the keynote speaker made a comparison between safety concerns in medicine and in aviation. At this moment, Goeltz writes, "a light of understanding started to glow in my mind."[17] Based on her decades of experience in a field in which preventing two airplanes from colliding — the ultimate systems error — was a task faced multiple times every day, she quickly grasped that clinical medicine similarly presented myriad opportunities for error and for error prevention. As a professional, she writes, "I began to understand how what happened to Mike could have occurred."[18] That is, she recognized that medical errors are not inexplicable aberrations, but they can be analyzed cognitively as systems failures and prevented through systems improvements. What she could not accept, as she told the audience at the conference, was the treatment of her family after her brother's death, the failure of *individuals* at the hospital, individuals who were members of the same community as her family, who worshipped beside them in church every Sunday, to speak to them with candor and compassion. Concerning her family's desire to achieve "forgiveness in our hearts," Goeltz writes: "It is difficult when no one will face us whom we can forgive."[19]

Roxanne Goeltz's experience of the aftermath of medical harm, and the connection she was able to make between the idiom and goals of her own profession and those of patient safety, became the catalyst for political action. She became a member of the National Patient Safety Foundation's Patient and Family Advisory Council and cofounded Consumers Advancing Patient Safety, an advocacy group that seeks to empower health care consumers to work in partnership with clinicians in preventing medical errors.[20] Other patients and family members have had similar conversion experiences, in which their devastating encounters with harmful medical mistakes have led them to make connections between the personal and the political, to organize and advocate for patient safety regionally and nationally, and, in particular, to collect and share stories of medical harm.[21] Organizations lobbying on behalf of patients' rights legislation, or to defeat tort reform proposals that would cap malpractice awards, are also making use of patients' and families' stories. The case of Linda McDougal, who was diagnosed with breast cancer and had a double mastectomy before her physicians realized her biopsy slide had been confused with that of another patient and that Mc-Dougal had never had cancer, became well known in 2003, when McDougal told her story in television advertisements that ran in seven states as part of a campaign to defeat tort reform legislation then pending in the U.S. Senate aimed at capping malpractice awards for pain and suffering.[22] Given that one stereotype of injured patients who sue doctors is of greedy litigants who, in the words of one physician interviewed about cases like McDougal's, "want to turn bad luck into good luck,"[23] stories of patients who survived but were grievously harmed by medical mistakes, told in their own words but shaped and deployed by activists, may challenge, or may harden, these stereotypes.

It is difficult to overstate how important the Internet is to the circulation of patients' and families' stories and to the ability of patients and families to learn about medical harm, to organize, and to share their own stories. Whereas in the fall of 1999 Roxanne Goeltz got one hit on a search for the phrase "medical error," a search on the same term in the fall of 2004 yielded 93,600 hits.[24] Web sites created by or for patients and families affected by medical mistakes may include stories, photos, video clips, memorials, chat rooms, self-help tips, PDFs (portable document format files), legislative updates, and many other resources. Then, there is the "Web documentary" that tells the story of Nancy Lim.[25]

Lim was a nurse-practitioner who, in the words of her husband, Michael Barnes, the creator of this Web site, "died from misdiagnosed complications from two surgeries to repair a botched Caesarean section."[26] During the Caesarean, Lim's bowel was perforated, resulting in a severe infection and, eventually, a temporary colostomy.[27] As in Jesse Rowe's case, the surgeries led to adhesions, scar tissue that can bind the intestines to the extent of compromising or destroying healthy tissue. Nine months after her son Max's birth, Lim experienced severe abdominal pain while at work; she consulted a colleague, also a clinician, who suspected a bowel obstruction, the choking of the intestines by an adhesion.[28] Barnes took Lim to the emergency room, where they told the admitting staff of the possibility of a bowel obstruction. Lim was diagnosed as having gallstones, received little monitoring overnight, and died the next morning of septic shock; a phlebotomist was the first to notice that she had stopped breathing. An autopsy confirmed that she died of a strangulating bowel obstruction and did not have gallstones. As Barnes writes, "She died even though she gave the emergency room an accurate diagnosis of her life-threatening condition."[29]

The full name of this Web site is "Blunt Instruments: Medicine, Law and the Death of Nancy Lim."[30] Barnes describes the twofold purpose of this Web site: "to tell the story of Nancy's death through the original documents" and "to create more awareness of how badly the legal and medical systems deal with incompetent doctors and hospitals."[31] The Web site contains more than 900 pages of scanned documents, including Lim's medical records, transcripts of depositions, personal and professional correspondence, and the newsletters that Barnes created to keep family and friends up to date on the investigation and lawsuit, and on his life as the single parent of Max. The site also includes dozens of captioned photos of Nancy and her family and friends, from childhood until shortly before her death at 41 years of age. It is difficult to imagine any other narrative form — an article, a book, a film, a gallery installation — that could contain this much material about one life and still be accessible to the "reader" attempting to explore it in a single encounter. The Web site is also alive, in that, a decade after Lim's death, Barnes was continuing to add "updates" in the form of article summaries and links relevant to medical error and patient safety.[32]

Readers of this narrative may find it useful to conceptualize the Web site as a private library dedicated to Nancy Lim, in which one can read the "original documents" relevant to her death and learn about her life through the photos and other permanent exhibitions. The narrator of this story seems to function as a librarian or curator: apart from telling us what the purpose of the collection is and how to find our way around, Michael Barnes seems to leave us to get on with our own research. However, this analogy will take us only so far. For the scholarly curator is also the author of many of the "original documents" he has assembled and is a character in others. In particular, he is the main character in his own deposition, which runs to 165 pages, and in which he tells the story of Nancy Lim's death in yet another way.[33]

One of the most emotionally wrenching parts of the story Barnes tells was elicited by a lawyer at deposition. Asked to describe his actions on the morning of his wife's death, Barnes tells of receiving a call "around 9:00 o'clock," from a nurse at the hospital, who informs him, "your wife has taken a turn for the worst."[34] He races to get dressed and find a babysitter: "And right before I had left the house, it occurred to me Nancy was in trouble. And before when she was in the hospital . . . I would take a picture with her and Max and leave her this picture. Then I would take Max home. As I was tearing out the door to go to the hospital . . . I grabbed the Polaroid, which was out of film — I had to get some film out of the refrigerator — took a picture of Max in the bouncy seat, stuck it in my pocket and drove to the hospital."[35] Barnes describes arriving at the hospital and being told that his wife had died: "And then Dr. Gardiner said something like you seem to be taking this okay. And then I said I have a nine-month-old baby to raise. I don't have any choice. And then Dr. Gardiner said how is Max doing? . . . I reached into my pocket and handed him the picture. He looked at the picture and smiled and gave it back to me."[36] The Polaroid that Michael Barnes took of Max on the morning his mother died is posted on the Web site.[37]

Michael Barnes's narrative persona as glimpsed in these documents is reminiscent of Sandra Gilbert's narrative persona in the story she tells. Like Gilbert, Barnes is a proud and loving spouse and parent, and a member of a large and devoted circle of family and friends that includes many health care professionals who are able to offer alternative readings of medical documents and ad hoc guidance throughout the investigation of the patient's death. Like Gilbert, he is a scholar who is deeply concerned about the fine details of the story he is both telling and enacting.[38] Both Barnes and Gilbert incorporate time lines, medical records, and legal transcripts and correspondence into their narratives; as scholars, they are accustomed to doing their research, documenting their sources, and getting their facts straight. Both combine linear and nonlinear methods of storytelling. Gilbert's dated, diary-like entries move back and forth in time, telling the story of her husband's death, but also many stories about his life, while Barnes's chosen form, the "Web documentary," is inherently nonlinear or, rather, encompasses multiple linear narratives. Both authors incorporate many photos of their spouses into their narratives, and both take pains to describe each of the ritual activities and sacred objects they rely on to honor the lives of their beloved partners or represent the lost loved one: Barnes holds onto his wife's old Honda, whereas Gilbert holds onto a Raggedy Andy doll, a good-luck gift from the family to Elliot before his surgery, "as if he were a life raft" (Gilbert 1997, 207).[39]

A further similarity exists between the stories told by Barnes and by Gilbert, a similarity that they share with the other authors of these personal and family narratives. In each story, the sense of personal and familial violation resulting from an incident of actual or suspected medical harm has a social dimension, represented by the violation of the covenantal relationship between an ill person and a health care institution. Before Elliot Gilbert's surgery, he would joke that "the Chair of Urology can't kill the Chair of English" (Gilbert 1997, 47). He and his surgeon were colleagues, after a fashion. After Elliot's death, Sandra Gilbert files suit against her own employer, the University of California, to claim the wages that Elliot Gilbert would have earned from the university had he not died as the result of an error made in a university medical center. Michael Barnes sues the hospital that employed Nancy Lim in one of its clinics to claim the wages that she would have earned had she not died as the result of an error made in this hospital. Carol Levine writes that as the result of her husband's injury she is "constantly vigilant" when any member of her family is hospitalized, "mindful of how little it takes to turn routine into disaster," although she has become able to "entrust" the hospital where the injury occurred with the continuing health care needs of her husband (Levine 2002, 241). Roxanne Goeltz describes the communal violation that occurred when the administrators of the local hospital failed to explain or express remorse for the death of a beloved community member. Given that residents of this small town may have few other health care options, the wound created by Mike's death may fail to heal, as family and friends are forced to rely on an institution that they regard as uncaring at best and suspect at worst. In describing how the failure of individuals and institutions to reach out to families in the immediate aftermath of a bad outcome can itself be experienced as a void that demands to be filled, Michael Rowe includes an excerpt from a conversation he had with his wife, Gail: "We want to be paid," she said, "And if we can't have Jesse back, we want to be paid in understanding, and if we can't have understanding then we want to be paid in money" (Rowe 2002, 235).

Physicians and medical students, coming across Jesse's stepmother's remark that if the family can't have their child back, and can't have "understanding," they want money, may well respond with cynicism: See, they admit it, they *really do* want to sue us, to destroy us. Any mention of "money" or litigation on the part of patients or families does tend to draw physicians' attention, but in every one of the narratives discussed in this chapter, patients and families are quite clear about why — and when — they consider or pursue litigation: to find out what happened, through depositions if disclosure was incomplete or badly handled; to secure compensation, through a litigated settlement if fair compensation was not offered following a known error that resulted in significant, permanent disability. "Money" is never the first thing on the minds of injured patients and their families, although it may well be the first thing on the minds of physicians. Doing close readings of these stories, in medical education, in grand rounds, or in similar settings, to draw students' and physicians' attention to what patients and families tell us that they need in the aftermath of medical harm, and to their varied reasons for considering litigation, may help physicians to distinguish between their own fears and stereotypes concerning "angry" patients and families and the reasonable expectations and concrete needs that these patients and families may have as the result of a medical mistake. Having gained some insight into the expectations and needs of patients and families, physicians may then be more willing and better equipped to take part in systemic efforts — implementing disclosure policies and practices, teaching students and physicians *how* to disclose and apologize for mistakes, developing fair compensation programs — aimed at meeting these expectations and needs.

Patients and families working with the National Patient Safety Foundation have identified, among the educational goals of the patient-safety movement, the need to "raise healthcare providers' awareness of the experiences of patients and their families and how they differ from the experiences of professionals who interact with the healthcare system on a regular basis."[40] Although this may be accomplished, as the National Patient Safety Foundation proposes, through the direct involvement of patients and families in patient-safety education — for example, as educators in medical school and continuing education programs on patient safety, and as members of patient and family advisory councils in hospitals[41] — the personal narratives of patients and families may also be effective teaching tools, in these and other contexts, in conveying the essential differences between how a mistake is experienced by a health care professional, within the context of a culture that is familiar to this professional, and by a health care consumer, within the context of an utterly alien culture. At the end of her book, Sandra Gilbert returns to that strange word used by her husband's surgeon, and reflects on what this single word may have revealed concerning the inability of this professional to tell her, and to tell himself, the truth about what happened to her husband:

> Remember what you said, Doctor . . . "For you, this is unpleasant, awful, I know. For *me*, it's shattering."
>
> And while your appraisal of *my* plight was curiously — how shall I put it? — *anesthetized*, you were certainly right about yourself. It was shattering. Perhaps too shattering to acknowledge? (Gilbert 2002, 337)

CHAPTER FOUR

Disclosure

There is basic intellectual agreement within the medical profession that telling patients the truth, including the truth about medical mistakes, constitutes a professional obligation for physicians. Since 1981, the Code of Medical Ethics of the American Medical Association (AMA) has included the following ethical opinion on truth telling:

> It is a fundamental ethical requirement that a physician should at all times deal honestly and openly with patients. Patients have a right to know their past and present medical status and to be free of any mistaken beliefs concerning their conditions. Situations occasionally occur in which a patient suffers significant medical complications that may have resulted from the physician's mistake or judgment. In these situations, the physician is ethically required to inform the patient of all the facts necessary to ensure understanding of what has occurred. Only through full disclosure is a patient able to make informed decisions regarding future medical care.
>
> . . . Concern regarding legal liability which might result following truthful disclosure should not affect the physician's honesty with a patient.[1]

Yet the nature of the practice of disclosure—what is *meant* by the phrase "telling the truth" in cases of medical error—continues to be among the most highly contested and emotionally fraught issues within conversations on patient safety in the United States and other developed nations. According to researchers who have closely examined physicians' attitudes toward disclosure, because physicians know that "truth telling has been the standard [of their profession] for many years," most will, if asked, "declare that they are always truthful with their patients."[2] These same physicians "may or may not" include the disclosure of medical mistakes as relevant to their own practice of truth telling.[3] The reasons for failing to disclose may depend, as philosopher Sissela Bok has argued in another context, on how one defines "truth telling" conceptually, or, as examples in the literature on medical error suggest, on self-deception or fear.[4] If physicians understand telling the truth narrowly as "not lying," when patients do not ask and physicians do not tell them about errors, physicians have not "lied" and there has been no breach of the truth-telling obligation. Some physicians may not be able to admit that they are capable of making errors, and so tell themselves and others that there was a "complication" or that the patient was "noncompliant." Or they do not investigate the possibility of error and take refuge in "not knowing" what happened—and thus have nothing to disclose. Finally, fear is often at the root of failure to disclose: If I disclose an error, the patient will sue me, ergo, I will not disclose errors.[5]

Medical educators are familiar with the ways in which the hidden curriculum, discussed in chapter 2, teaches students and residents how to think and talk about their own mistakes and those of their colleagues. Observing more senior physicians, students learn that their mentors and supervisors believe in, practice, and reward the concealment of errors. They learn how to talk about unanticipated outcomes until a "mistake" morphs into a "complication." Above all, they learn not to tell the patient anything. Given the depth of physicians' resistance to disclosure and the lengths to which some will go to justify the habit of nondisclosure—it was only a technical error, things just happen, the patient won't understand, the patient does not need to know—there is a pressing need for fresh conceptual tools that can help physicians confront and change deeply entrenched beliefs, fears, and practices, and to weigh their moral and professional obligations, including their obligations to the next generation of physicians, against their terror of being found out, humiliated, and destroyed. The preceding three chapters proposed ways to use personal narratives about medical mistakes as tools for exploring physicians' obligations and patients' and families' expectations in the aftermath of medical harm. This chapter will explore a little-known essay by Dietrich Bonhoeffer, together with the historical circumstances of this essay's composition, as a text on disclosure, and suggest how the text may constitute a further resource both for understanding what is meant by telling the truth and for overcoming the powerful temptation to avoid doing so.

The Text in Context

In a letter to his friend Eberhard Bethge in mid-November 1943, Dietrich Bonhoeffer writes that he has drafted an "an essay on 'What is "speaking the truth"?' "[6] Bonhoeffer was then seven months into his confinement at the military prison in the Tegel district of Berlin, where he was being held on suspicion of involvement in a plot to overthrow Hitler, a plot in which he and his family were deeply involved. Two subsequent letters to Bethge again mention the essay and its subject. In his authoritative biography of Bonhoeffer, Bethge describes the circumstances of Bonhoeffer's life during the composition of this essay. "Bonhoeffer's period at Tegel was filled by his stubborn but successful efforts to conceal the true facts. His family and friends helped him weave an intricate net of camouflage . . . which held until after the catastrophe of 20 July 1944," when a failed assassination attempt against Hitler revealed the "true facts" of the conspiracy.[7] During the early months of his imprisonment, Bonhoeffer was regularly interrogated by military judge Manfred Roeder while simultaneously exchanging encoded messages with his family so that he knew what he could safely disclose and what he needed to conceal to protect the conspiracy and individual conspirators. According to Bethge:

> During the period of interrogation Bonhoeffer used up a lot of paper in his cell writing drafts of letters to Roeder, in which he supplemented or corrected his statements after a hearing. Roeder had occasionally encouraged him to make these notes, and Bonhoeffer seized the opportunity to gain time and ponder how to build the edifice of his stories further. The notes that have been preserved give a fairly exact picture of what was at stake in this tiny corner of the resistance's fight, the way in which Bonhoeffer defended himself and concealed the real facts of the conspiracy, what he produced and what he suppressed. His fragmentary essay, "What Is Meant by 'Telling the Truth'?" emerged during these months, and the notes reveal something of the true background of that study. Their confusing content mercilessly shows the consequences of the conspirators' struggle. The fact that Bon-

hoeffer wrote his essay in those weeks shows how much he was aware of his dilemma, and that he did not seek to pretend or hide anything from himself.[8]

What Bethge describes as a "fragmentary" work based on "confusing" source material has perplexed scholars and other readers. Philosopher Jean Bethke Elshtain, who devoted considerable attention to this essay in an article on "Bonhoeffer and Modernity," acknowledges that "many" readers "find [it] so enigmatic."[9] Sissela Bok quotes from the essay and includes a lengthy excerpt from it in the appendix to *Lying,* her influential study of "moral choice in public and private life," but does not offer any analysis of it.[10] Nor is the essay a frequent subject of commentary among Bonhoeffer scholars writing in English. Contemporary English-speaking readers may be further confused by the current location of this essay within the Bonhoeffer canon in translation, where it has traditionally been appended to *Ethics* — Elshtain, for example, describes it as "the fragment on truth with which *Ethics* concludes" — instead of being framed contextually by inclusion within collections of the prison writings.[11]

Admittedly, "fragmentary" and "enigmatic" are not usually what one looks for in a conceptual tool, particularly one derived from an apparently "religious" source. Moreover, it is fair to ask how Bonhoeffer's reflection on and justification of his own practice of *non*disclosure and outright deception may inform efforts not only to promote truth telling following medical harm but also to support efforts to define "what is meant by telling the truth" as the practice of *full* disclosure, namely, offering injured patients and their families a complete and truthful account of what happened, why it happened, and who is accountable for preventing future harm, plus an apology and fair compensation.[12] Yet a case can be made for applying this unusual essay, written under unusual circumstances, to the all-too-common problem of nondisclosure, a problem that poses a barrier to all other efforts to make justice for injured patients and their families, and also to attend adequately to the needs and fears of physicians. First, Bonhoeffer's insistence on framing truth telling as a practice embedded in human relationships and social contexts is useful in thinking about defining and changing "what is meant by telling the truth" within the complex amalgam of people, technology, market forces, and attendant values that constitute the culture of the contemporary hospital. Second, the tension between individual and authority that is expressed throughout the essay is an important factor in the uneasy relationship between physicians who may unintentionally injure patients and the hospitals where these injuries occur. Third, the themes presented in this essay are linked to other important themes in Bonhoeffer's writings — in particular, the "view from below" as ethical standpoint and "responsibility" as ethical norm — that are germane to the ethics of the aftermath of medical harm, but are here highlighted in terms of the responsible action on which all subsequent actions will turn: telling the truth.

The Murderer at the Door: Bonhoeffer's Critique of Kant

Although the immediate circumstances of his interrogation in 1943 prompted Bonhoeffer to draft his essay on truth telling — which is referred to hereafter as the "Tegel essay" — a well-known section of his *Ethics*, drafted before his imprisonment, anticipates the arguments that he will make in the Tegel essay and identifies Kant as his principal philosophical foil.[13] In the section on "Conscience," Bonhoeffer writes:

> From the principle of truthfulness Kant draws the grotesque conclusion that I must even return an honest "yes" to the enquiry of the murderer who breaks into my house and asks whether my friend whom he is pursuing has taken refuge there; in such a case self-righteousness of conscience has become outrageous presumption and blocks the path of responsible action. Responsibility is the total and realistic response of man to the claim of God and of our neighbor; but this example shows in its true light how the response of a conscience which is bound by principles is only a partial one.[14]

Bonhoeffer refers to the same Kantian principle in a footnote to the Tegel essay: "Kant, of course, declared that he was too proud ever to utter a falsehood; indeed he unintentionally carried this principle *ad absurdum* by saying that he would feel himself obliged to give truthful information even to a criminal looking for a friend of his who had concealed himself in his house" (363n1). The offending passage is found in Kant's essay, "On a Supposed Right to Lie from Altruistic Motives," in which he refutes the notion of the "benevolent lie," the falsehood told to protect another.[15] For Kant, truthfulness is "a duty which must be regarded as the ground of all duties" and a "sacred and absolutely commanding decree of reason, limited by no expediency."[16] The likelihood, even the certainty, that one person's truth telling will result in another person being unjustly harmed does not, for Kant, have any bearing on the principle.[17]

Bonhoeffer's initial engagement with this text comes, as noted, in the context of a discussion of conscience. Writing from the perspective of a society in which the good, that is, loyal, citizen says, " 'My conscience is Adolf Hitler,' "

Bonhoeffer argues against any idea of conscience that takes compliance with immanence — whether in the form of a human being, a civic law, or religion — as its sole or primary reference point (239). Bonhoeffer can say of himself that "Jesus Christ has become my conscience" not merely as a way of rejecting the loathsome rhetoric of Nazism, but because a conscience that is identified with Christ is a conscience that is actively allied with the interests of the neighbor (240). Having proclaimed this dual allegiance to "the living God and the living man as he confronts me in Jesus Christ," Bonhoeffer then takes on Kant, in the famous passage on "responsibility" (240).

In Nazi Germany, the murderer at the door and the friend hiding in the house were neither extreme nor hypothetical cases, but concrete realities. To betray the friend to the murderer in either the name of Christian conscience or the name of the categorical imperative was a "grotesque" misunderstanding of *why* we should tell the truth. We should not do so out of loyalty to abstract principle: As Bonhoeffer tells us at the beginning of his *Ethics*, the "villain and the saint" both tend to transgress rather than be contained by ethical systems (66). We should not do so to keep our consciences pure: This places us on the same moral footing as the Nazi functionary, his conscience aligned with evil, who demands, in the name of the law, that we tell the truth about where our friend is hiding.

Having radically detached the practice of truth telling from the ethical tautology that one ought to tell the truth because telling the truth is (always) the right thing to do, Bonhoeffer identifies the *reason* that we tell the truth, or undertake any action that we define as ethical: to be responsible, to demonstrate our "total and realistic response . . . to the claim of God and of our neighbor." In the context of this discussion of conscience, the neighbor is the other who is in "concrete distress" (241). In "the view from below," a passage usually appended to "After Ten Years," Bonhoeffer's moral "reckoning" of the anti-Nazi resistance at the end of 1942, he is even more specific about the identity of the neighbor, who is the "outcast, the suspects, the maltreated, the powerless, the oppressed, the reviled — in short . . . those who suffer."[18] Our moral responsibility, whether or not we frame it in terms of Christian ethics, is to learn how to see the world from "the perspective of those who suffer" and to respond.[19]

We can now turn to the Tegel essay itself, which Bethge has contextualized historically as Bonhoeffer's reflection on the experience of being ordered to tell the (factual) truth about his knowledge of the conspiracy and of his efforts to tell the (moral) truth by maintaining his responsibility toward those already harmed by the regime and those who would be harmed should Bonhoeffer and his fellow prisoners reveal the facts. An intertextual perspective on this essay, mindful of its close thematic relationship to the "Conscience" material in *Ethics*, might describe the difference between the two texts thus: Whereas in "Conscience," Bonhoeffer is concerned with the morality of truth telling, in the Tegel essay he is concerned with the epistemology of truth telling. What do we *mean* by the phrase "telling the truth"? What is the nature of this practice?

Bonhoeffer begins his essay by announcing his project and charting truth telling as a practice embedded in the parent-child relationship. Because we are taught from earliest childhood both that we must speak the truth to our parents and that we cannot demand that our parents speak the truth to us, we quickly learn that " 'telling the truth' means something different according to the particular situation in which one stands. Account must be taken of one's relationships at each particular time. The question must be asked whether and in what way a [person] is entitled to demand truthful speech of others."[20] From the start, Bonhoeffer rejects any theologizing of the categorical imperative. Although Christians do owe God the truth, "God is not a general principle, but the living God who has set me in a living life and who demands service of me within the living life."[21] To refuse to acknowledge the earthly, relational context of truth *telling* is to treat Christ as a "metaphysical idol."[22] Rather, "the truthfulness which we owe to God must assume a concrete form in the world."[23] Because all relationships, all contexts, are not identical, telling the truth is neither a reflex nor "solely a matter of moral character"[24] — ". . . it is also a matter of correct appreciation of real situations and of serious reflection upon them. The more complex the actual situations of a man's life, the more responsible and the more difficult will be his task of 'telling the truth' . . . the ethical cannot be detached from reality, and consequently continual progress in learning to appreciate reality is a necessary ingredient in ethical action. In the question with which we are now concerned, action consists of speaking."[25]

In other words, Kant had not anticipated the complex reality of Nazism. At a certain level, of course, Bonhoeffer agrees with Kant. Ideally, individuals and society ought to be in accordance, and the categorical imperative becomes a way of describing the ethics of civil society. As theologian Robin W. Lovin points out with respect to the politics of Bonhoeffer and his fellow conspirators: "The goals of these plotters were for the most part frankly restorationist. The aim was not a new social order for Germany, but the revival of the forms of government that would make stability and peace possible . . . Bonhoeffer's writings during the War years reflect the language and ideas of the German conservatism that became the center of wartime resistance."[26]

Thus, Bonhoeffer, a political conservative and lover of truth, memorably asserts in *Ethics* that "it is worse for a liar to tell the truth than of a lover of truth to lie."[27] Translated into the ethics of interrogation, it is worse for a judicial representative of a genocidal regime to demand that Bonhoeffer reveal the facts of the conspiracy than it is for Bonhoeffer to conceal these facts. The interrogator lies by demanding the truth in the name of injustice; the prisoner tells the truth by refusing to enter into an illegitimate truth-telling relationship.

How Can I Speak the Truth?

One of the many challenges in implementing and upholding truth-telling practices after medical mistakes, including reporting errors to authorities inside and outside the hospital as well as disclosing errors to patients and families, is that physicians may not view truth-seeking efforts within hospitals as legitimate, even if these efforts are carried out with the laudable goal of wanting to make hospitals safer for patients rather than simply in an effort to "blame and shame" those deemed "responsible" for a given error. Despite evidence from some health care institutions that strongly suggests a correlation between the practice of full disclosure and reduced risks and costs associated with litigation, many physicians remain convinced that full disclosure is intended merely to deflect lawsuits away from institutions and toward individuals.[28] In such a fearful, suspicious environment, might a physician believe that Bonhoeffer is offering moral shelter for the practice of nondisclosure, even of lying, to protect one's self or one's peers?[29]

Perhaps, but this would be a grave misreading of Bonhoeffer, whose goal in not disclosing a factual account of the conspiracy to his interrogators was not self-preservation, but the protection of the conspiracy's efforts to jam "a spoke in the wheel" of Nazism and, in so doing, to honor the "the perspective of those who suffer."[30] Physicians are expected to honor this perspective as a professional obligation. As Albert Wu argues, "a physician's responsibility to disclose a mistake to a patient can be derived from the fiduciary character of the doctor-patient relationship" and from the principles of biomedical ethics: "A physician's obligation to respect patient autonomy indicates that a doctor has an ethical obligation to disclose mistakes to patients."[31] A hospital exists to care for the sick, whose perspective is, by definition, that of "those who suffer." A patient who is injured in the course of caregiving suffers twice; this patient is doubly vulnerable within the institution, whose culture perceives this patient as a potential legal adversary, a "risk" to be "managed." A physician who has injured a patient by making a mistake and seeks to avoid disclosing this error, and thus to deny justice to the one who suffers, is offered no moral shelter by Bonhoeffer, whose essay on truth telling concludes with the following rubric:

> How can I speak the truth?
>
> a By perceiving who causes me to speak and what entitles me to speak.
>
> b By perceiving the place at which I stand.
>
> c By relating to this context the object about which I am making some assertion.[32]

The physician who is contemplating the disclosure of medical error should perceive that the "fiduciary character of the doctor-patient relationship" causes and entitles him to speak if he has injured a patient through error. He should perceive his standpoint as that of a responsible and compassionate caregiver, as well as with reference to the bioethical principles that, for him, constitute professional obligations. Although Bonhoeffer objects to an uncritical adherence to principles, without any reference to reality, he surely believes in professional ethics, the obligations that one is bound to carry out while performing a legitimate professional role, as this Tegel conversation, reported by a fellow prisoner, makes clear: "When we took our walk together . . . every day, we spoke of political, religious and scientific problems . . . He also spoke of the tragic fate of the German people, whose qualities and shortcomings he knew. He told me that it was very difficult for him to desire its defeat, but it was necessary . . . He stated that *as a pastor* it was his duty not just to comfort the victims of the man who drove down a busy street like a maniac, but to try to stop him."[33]

Returning to the hypothetical physician who is contemplating the disclosure of a medical mistake, professional obligations and the nature of his caregiving relationship to his patient may not be sufficient motivators for him to acknowledge an ethical standpoint that identifies full disclosure as the responsible course of action following harm. In the course of alleviating suffering, he has caused suffering, yet, due to his professional status and the norms of his professional culture, he may have to make a conscious effort to see the situation "from below," from the patient's perspective. As Bonhoeffer writes in the passage appended to "After Ten Years," in his description of the "view from below" as ethical standpoint, "we have to learn that personal suffering is a more effective key, a more rewarding principle for exploring the world in thought and action than personal good fortune."[34] As long as the physician cannot see that the patient's suffering, and *not his own suffering*, constitutes the "view from below"; as long as he cannot admit that *he* is not the sole or principal victim of this incident due to its perceived impact on his career, income, or self-image; as long as he fears what the injured patient might do to him rather than recognizing disclosure as part of the narrative of caregiving, he will not be able to understand and embrace full disclosure as an ethical norm.

This hypothetical physician is not alone in his discomfort. Telling the truth is hard, and changing the norms of professional and institutional culture from nondisclosure to disclosure is even harder. To effect this cultural shift, there will be a need for stories that offer not merely "ethics lessons" — physicians already know that they are supposed to tell the truth and already believe that they do tell the truth — but also attest to the psychological and spiritual anguish that may attach itself to truth telling and concealment, which Bethge captures when he describes Bonhoeffer's interrogation notes as both "confusing" and "merciless."

When physicians talk about a story that changed the way they thought about truth telling following medical error, they frequently mention "The Chief of Medicine," physician Howard Brody's retelling of "The Grand Inquisitor" episode in *The Brothers Karamazov*.[35] In Brody's retelling, the Christ figure is represented by a medical student who, having witnessed a procedure that "went badly," decides, in violation of the hidden curriculum and the orders of the physicians in charge of the case, to tell the patient's family that the patient is dying.[36] Her interrogation by the Grand Inquisitor figure, represented by the hospital's Chief of Medicine, reveals, again and again, how frightening and bewildering an error can be to individual physicians as it unfolds. Reading this story, physicians recognize in themselves the idealistic student who believes that the "perspective of those who suffer" belongs first to the patient. They also recognize the "horrified" internists who "had made a terrible hash of things" and were "terrified of malpractice suits," but who, in refusing to tell the patient and family what had happened, were "acting so as to maximize the chances that they would be sued."[37] And they recognize, in the Chief of Medicine, both the idolatry and the fragility of power; the Chief is terrified of disclosing errors because he is terrified of the consequences of revealing to patients that physicians are human.

There is room in the culture of medicine for another rich, provocative, theologically informed story about truth telling, and Bonhoeffer's fragmentary, enigmatic little essay, and the circumstances of its composition, is such a story. As a conceptual tool that takes the psychological and spiritual as well as the moral dimensions of truth telling seriously, the Tegel essay may speak to physicians in much the same way that Brody's retelling of Dostoevsky has. And knowledge of the essay's historical context may move physicians toward a reassessment of and reconciliation with their own truth-telling obligations toward the "neighbor" whom they have inadvertently harmed.

For, after all, they are *not* Dietrich Bonhoeffer in Tegel Prison, and the injured patient — or even his malpractice attorney — is *not* Manfred Roeder.

CHAPTER FIVE

Apology

At the outset of any discussion involving those troublesome words "I'm sorry," one ought always to make a commonsense distinction: To say "I'm sorry your father died" is not at all the same thing as saying, "I'm sorry I killed your father." When these two statements are juxtaposed in this way, we immediately recognize that the former is an expression of sympathy concerning an event in which the speaker was not necessarily involved in any way, whereas the latter is an expression of responsibility, an apology for an event in which the speaker was intimately involved. Too often, however, when physicians, academics, journalists, lawyers, or policymakers talk about whether, when, and how the words "I'm sorry" should be spoken in the aftermath of medical harm, this crucial distinction is blurred, and "I'm sorry your father died" — sympathy, no more — is forced to stand in for "I'm sorry I made a mistake that killed your father" — a true apology.

This chapter examines the question of apology after medical harm within the context of the current trend in many states to craft and adopt "I'm sorry" laws, which offer varying degrees of legal protection for expressions of sympathy and even admissions of fault after incidents of harm, including medical mistakes. Although this trend has been the subject of influential articles in legal journals and has been addressed in professional journals with reference to the role of apology in the mediation process, it is not always well known or well understood among health care professionals, health care ethicists, and other nonlawyers who are interested in patient safety.[1] Two of the most recently enacted "I'm sorry" laws — in Colorado and Oregon, both of which passed their laws in 2003 — were specifically designed to protect physicians and, in Colorado, other health care professionals as well, who apologize after making medical mistakes. As a result, scholars and professionals grappling with the role of apology after medical mistakes need to understand this legal and policy trend, particularly with respect to its ethical implications for the just treatment of injured patients and their families.

The words "I'm sorry" and the nature of the proper relationship between persons after one person has injured another have a rich history of associations within religious tradition; some of these associations are explored in this book in chapter 7. Jonathan Cohen and Lee Taft, two of the most influential legal commentators on the "I'm sorry" laws, whose analyses are discussed in this chapter, have theological competency that informs their consideration of the psychological and cultural meanings of an apology, in addition to its legal definition.[2] Other commentators, such as the legal theorist Martha Minow, who has written about South Africa's Truth and Reconciliation Commission and other efforts to rebuild societies after genocide, war crimes, and other profoundly destabilizing events, acknowledge the impact that religious language and practices, including the language of apology and forgiveness, may have in the ostensibly secular realms of law and policy in civil society.[3] The willingness of legal scholars to examine the meaning of apology in religious discourse and in related secular practices when assessing the nature of apology — in particular, about whether there is or ought to be such a thing as a "safe" or consequence-free apology — suggests that it is unwise to equivocate in the matter of apology, to argue that by meeting a legal or technical definition one has satisfied a deeply rooted psychological or cultural expectation. It also suggests that insight into the religious and cultural nuances of this practice may be integral to understanding what is meant by the words "I'm sorry," how these words are related to actions, past, present, and future, and what these words and actions convey to the person who has been harmed.[4]

The "I'm Sorry" Laws

In his article "Legislating Apology: The Pros and Cons," Jonathan Cohen, the University of Florida legal scholar whose work on apology has been particularly influential in legal and policy circles, defines apology as "an admission of one's fault combined with an expression of regret for having injured another as well as an expression of sympathy for the other's injury."[5] He underscores the revolutionary nature of the "I'm sorry" law trend by pointing out that apologies, under American law, have been viewed as "evidence of liability": Say you're sorry, and this statement, under the law, could indeed be used against you.[6] Although there are exceptions to this rule—Cohen cites mediation and settlement negotiations as legal forums in which apologies have long been encouraged—and although injured persons have long made clear that *not* receiving an apology contributes to the anger that triggers lawsuits, physicians' reluctance to apologize for their mistakes, and hospital lawyers' and risk managers' advice to avoid such apologies, have, in part, been based on this legal precedent. In his article, which was published prior to the adoption of the medical malpractice-specific Colorado and Oregon laws, Cohen outlines laws and pending legislation, plus related case law, in more than a dozen states. He identifies the conceptual definitions of apology, and their ethical and legal implications, operative in these proposed and actual laws as follows[7]:

- "I'm sorry" as sympathy; admission of fault not protected by law

These versions of the "I'm sorry" laws, which have been enacted in Texas (1999), California (2000), Florida (2001), Washington (2002), and Tennessee (2002), protect expressions of "sympathy or a general sense of benevolence"[8] after an accident resulting in injury or death. However, if the person responsible for the accident admits fault as part of the same "benevolent gesture"—"I'm so sorry, I feel terrible that you were hurt, it was my fault!"—or at another time, the admission of fault itself ("It was my fault!") is not protected and could be used as evidence of liability in a lawsuit.

- "I'm sorry" as sympathy, with full apology possibly protected by law

The first "I'm sorry" law was enacted in Massachusetts (1986)[9] at the instigation of a state legislator who was dismayed and angered when he did not receive an apology from the driver of a car that had hit and killed his young daughter. When he learned that the driver wanted to apologize but had been warned against doing so by his lawyer, the legislator sought to protect the statement that the driver wanted to make, and that he, the grieving father, wanted to receive, from being used as evidence against the driver.[10] Versions of this law are currently under consideration in Illinois, Iowa, Rhode Island, and West Virginia.[11] The Massachusetts statute is silent on whether an admission of fault—integral to a true apology as opposed to a mere expression of sympathy—would or would not be protected from being used as evidence of liability.

- "I'm sorry" as apology: admission of fault explicitly protected by law

Colorado's version of the "I'm sorry" law, which was passed in April 2003, explicitly protects statements of fault, as well as expressions of sympathy, from being used as evidence of liability.[12] Oregon's 2003 law protects both "expressions of regret" and "apology," with the latter presumably including fault-admitting statements.[13] Pending bills in Connecticut and Hawaii appear to offer similar protection for admissions of fault.[14] The Connecticut bill does so by eschewing the use of "benevolent gestures" language and stating simply that "apology" is protected,[15] whereas the Hawaii bill distinguishes between "benevolent gestures" and "apologies" and protects both statements.[16]

With respect to case law, appeals courts in Georgia and Vermont have issued decisions in medical malpractice cases that offer some legal protection for benevolent gestures or fault-admitting apologies. In the Georgia case,[17] the court ruled that an offer of financial assistance following a medical injury was not itself evidence of liability and declared that "actions made on the impulse of benevolence or sympathy should be encouraged" rather than used as grounds for litigation. In the Vermont cases,[18] courts ruled that fault-admitting apologies by physicians were not in and of themselves sufficient to meet the standard three-part test for determining negligence.

Because medical malpractice cases are won or lost based on this three-part test, and because physicians, patients, commentators, and the public frequently misconstrue what "negligence" means in a legal context, a brief description of the three-part test may be helpful. It is important to keep in mind that "negligence" is a legal term, not a medical term. A harmful mistake, even a mistake that results in the death of a patient, can be described as "negligence" only if it meets the three-part test: (1) there was a departure from a recognized standard of care, (2) the patient was harmed, and (3) the harm was the result of the departure from the standard of care. The standard of care for abdominal surgeries, for example, may include inadvertent perforations of organs. Such perforations may lead to infection, the need for further surgeries, even death: The cases of Jesse Rowe and Nancy Lim, discussed in chapter 3, involve injuries of this kind. These technical errors, although undeniably harmful, do not constitute negligence in the legal sense of the word, because they do not meet the three-part test. A patient or a surviving family member would not win a malpractice judgment in such a case, and might be advised, as were Rowe's and Lim's families, that they should not even attempt to bring such a case.[19] However, it is also important to keep in mind that medical harm is *harm*, even if it is not the result of "negligence," that is to say, the result of substandard care or "bad" doctors. Therefore, harmful mistakes or other unintentional injuries that occur *within* the standard of care must be disclosed to patients, who have the right to this crucial information about their health. Such patients should also receive fair compensation for medical or financial needs resulting from the harm. The next chapter discusses several programs that do precisely this: provide fair compensation without litigation.

As noted, apart from the case-law examples, only the Colorado and Oregon "I'm sorry" laws are specifically concerned with medical mistakes. The other statutes and proposed legislation speak more generally about "accidents," and legislators in at least two states, Massachusetts and Connecticut, were evidently thinking about automotive accidents — protecting the driver who blurts out "I'm sorry" or even "I'm sorry, it was my fault" from being sued based solely on this statement — when they crafted their versions of the "I'm sorry" laws.[20] These laws share the goal of reducing lawsuits of all kinds, but Jonathan Cohen, writing before the adoption of the Colorado and Oregon laws, makes an important distinction between medical mistakes and fender benders. Although drivers involved in an accident probably do not have any prior relationship with one another, physicians and patients almost always do, and "the need for apologies [is] greatest when the parties have a prior relationship."[21] Hence his observation that it is the failure to apologize, *not the accident itself,* that leads to "relational breakdown" and thence to lawsuits, when the injured party is insulted by the lack of concern, compassion, and accountability on the part of the person who, while caring for him, caused the injury (Cohen 2002, 843). As Cohen memorably writes, "Accidentally injuring another makes one a klutz. Failing to apologize makes one a jerk." Thus, although policymakers in most states may not have had medical mistakes in mind when crafting these laws, they are arguably especially relevant in this context, in which apology, or the failure to apologize, may profoundly affect the nature of the relationship between physician and patient.

Media coverage of the "I'm sorry" laws has frequently confused the two senses of the phrase "I'm sorry" by characterizing the legal protection of expressions of sympathy, common to all these laws, as legal protection for "apologies," a word that, when used in these laws, tends to be reserved for admissions of fault.[22] (Thus, one commentator, writing in a professional journal for physicians, states that California's "I'm sorry" law protects "apologies but not specific admissions of fault,"[23] when in fact California's law does not use the word "apologies.") This point is of more than semantic interest. Whenever the definition of "apology" is reduced to the totemic phrase "I'm sorry," whether by journalists, lawyers, mediators, or physicians, accountability — *mea culpa, my fault* — is reduced to mere regret: I am sorry that something terrible happened to you, let's move on. We will explore these critiques of the "I'm sorry" law trend, and of instrumental approaches to apology in the context of dispute resolution, at a later point.

The Oregon and Colorado "I'm Sorry" Laws: Context and Content

Oregon's "I'm sorry" law, House Bill 3361, was sponsored at the request of the Oregon Medical Association. It protects "any expression of regret or apology made by or on behalf of" anyone licensed by the state's Board of Medical Examiners—a physician. The law is retroactive, applying to apologies made prior to 2003, unless a judgment has already been rendered in a case. It prevents an apology or similar statement from being cited as evidence of liability in administrative hearings, mediation, or arbitration, as well as in civil lawsuits. Unlike Colorado's law, it is not specifically concerned with apologies after "unanticipated outcomes" of medical treatment, but more broadly protects apologies in the context of "any civil action" against a licensed physician. Media commentators characterized the bill as being part of the medical association's tort-reform agenda; the legislative sponsor described it as conducive to physician-patient communications, whereas a plaintiff's attorney interviewed disagreed: "When you make a mistake, you're man enough to own up to it . . . You don't try to find some refuge where you're not held accountable . . . the doctor's association wants that to be buried. That's not the right thing."[24]

Colorado's "I'm sorry" law, House Bill 1232, is described in two ways by COPIC, a Denver-based insurer that provides malpractice coverage to nearly six thousand physicians regionally and that was instrumental in the passage of this law.[25] (COPIC's own compensation program for patients injured by physicians it insures is discussed in the next chapter.) In its summary of the legislative victory, COPIC describes the law as "protecting the patient-physician relationship" and, more broadly, as "tort reform." Patient-safety advocates may find these goals difficult to approach simultaneously or may even bridle at their being linked. At a time when physicians' sometimes vitriolic rhetoric over insurance rates and "frivolous" lawsuits may smear "greedy" patients as well as malpractice insurers and personal-injury lawyers, the rallying cry of "tort reform" would appear to have little to do with the "patient-physician relationship." COPIC connects the two issues by quoting a physician who testified in support of the Colorado bill: "Injured patients expect and deserve an explanation. They want to know what went wrong, and they want to be assured that steps are being taken to prevent similar occurrences to others. Yet [physicians'] fear of exposure to the tort system can act as a powerful deterrent to this communication."[26]

HB 1232 seeks to remedy this problem by protecting, in any situation involving an unanticipated medical outcome or in arbitration related to such a situation, "any and all statements, affirmations, gestures, or conduct expressing apology, fault, sympathy, commiseration, condolence, compassion, or a general sense of benevolence which are made by a health care provider or an employee of a health care provider" to an injured patient or her family or other representative.[27] Although some of the language — the words "sympathy" and "benevolence" — is also included in the other "I'm sorry" laws, the Colorado bill contains much that is truly different. "Fault" is explicitly protected, even to the extent of using that word in addition to "apology." Protection is extended to health care institutions and their employees, rather than being limited to the individual who made the mistake, and the protected communication covers statements made to persons other than the injured patient. As COPIC points out, HB 1232 does not offer immunity from malpractice suits, but "only to prevent the statement [of sympathy, apology, fault, etc.] itself from being used"[28] as evidence of liability or negligence.

The reaction to affording such broad protections to apologies after medical mistakes has been mixed. The Colorado Patient Safety Coalition, a consumer group, supported HB 1232, suggesting that patients and patient safety advocates did not view the measure solely in terms of tort reform benefiting physicians and insurers, but also as a means of addressing some of the needs of injured patients and their families — in this case, their needs for apology, disclosure, and accountability. However, a columnist for the *Denver Post* characterized the law as " 'sorry' protection": "if doctors want to tell patients that they are sorry for their mistakes, then they ought to be prepared to live with the consequences . . . What other professionals have this sort of protection?"[29]

This commentator makes several common errors and overstatements, conflating medical mistakes with deliberate fraud and using extreme examples ("Sorry, I hacked off your leg") without explaining that the "I'm sorry" law does not protect physicians from being sued, but only protects the apology statement itself from being used as evidence. In particular, wrong-site surgery — hacking off the wrong leg, removing the wrong kidney — is a textbook example of the three-part legal test for negligence: a departure from the standard of care; a harm to the patient; a causal link between the error and the harm. A hospital would be inclined to settle such a clear-cut case quickly, because there would be ample evidence that could be uncovered by the patient's counsel regardless of whether the negligent surgeon made any statement. Contrary to the columnist's example, an apology in such a case would not offer "absolution without messy legal entanglements," because a surgeon who performed wrong-site surgery would likely face disciplinary action.[30]

Apology as Responsible Action

Nevertheless, this commentator's point, that apologies ought to have consequences, is also raised by Lee Taft, a former plaintiff's attorney who is highly critical of what he terms "the commodification of apology,"[31] which he detects in the "I'm sorry" statutes and in certain alternatives to litigation, such as mediation. Like Jonathan Cohen, who describes the failure to apologize after harm as "morally offensive,"[32] Taft views apology as a moral act, "because it acknowledges the existence of right and wrong and confirms that a norm of right behavior has been broken."[33] Although Cohen cautiously supports legal and policy efforts to protect so-called "safe" apologies as a means of promoting the repair of relationships damaged by accidental harm — and insists that, with respect to medical mistakes, physicians who make mistakes must disclose them, as a professional obligation[34] — Taft believes that the "I'm sorry" law trend toward protecting apologies "subverts a moral process."[35] An apology may consist of words, but it is not merely words, a formula that repairs all broken relations and offers magical protection against litigation. Rather, according to Taft, it is an act that the offender must understand to be risky, because it requires the sincere acknowledgment of having done wrong: *mea culpa, my fault*. And it is an act that the injured party must understand to be risky (not safe, not formulaic), so that it can be recognized and accepted as meaningful, respectful, and worthy of response. Though Taft's critique was published before the advent of "I'm sorry" laws specifically designed to protect fault-admitting apologies after medical mistakes, he anticipates the laws by imagining how a "safe" statement after medical error might sound: "how would you respond if the negligent doctor said only, 'I'm sorry you are suffering?' Would an expression of sympathy devoid of accountability help you heal? Would the protected words restore the moral balance between you and the doctor?"[36]

Clinicians and others may reject, resist, or be unable to comprehend the idea that an unintentional medical injury — in particular, one that does not result from negligence but occurs within the standard of care—might fall into the category of moral transgression, if only because it is impossible to eliminate human error from the practice of medicine. According to human factors research, which examines the role of human actions in systems errors, even the best trained, most attentive workers will regularly make errors of omission, the skipped steps in familiar routines that constitute "the single largest category of human performance problems," whereas such workers will also occasionally make errors of commission, performing routine actions incorrectly.[37] Thus, "thou shalt not make errors of omission or commission" is not enforceable as a moral code or as a matter of practice. It is an axiom of ethics that "ought implies can": People should not be held to standards they can not possibly meet. So, although physicians may at some level *feel* morally culpable when their actions harm their patients—and physicians' autobiographical accounts of their own mistakes, as well as research into the psychological impact of medical error on physicians, strongly indicate that this is the case for many in the profession—they may simultaneously argue that patients are occasionally harmed by even the most conscientious of practitioners, that the physician is not in control of every aspect of a patient's care, that mistakes sometimes just *happen*.

Nevertheless, recalling "ought implies can," the physician who may resist or reject the idea that medical mistakes are moral wrongs—and this would seem to be a defensible position with respect to mistakes that do not constitute negligence, the conscious violation of acknowledged standards—ought to be able to grasp Cohen's and Taft's point concerning the morality of apology *after* mistakes. In Cohen's words, failing to apologize, after *any* harm to another person, makes one a jerk. Only a jerk would fail to apologize after injuring another person, would fail to acknowledge the suffering, whether physical, financial, or emotional, that resulted from the mistake, would fail to acknowledge that the mistake did not "happen" only to the person who made it.

Another kind of jerk, the cynical kind, mouths the "safe" words, the ones that he's been told patients want to hear, the ones that will inoculate him against a lawsuit, but he commits himself neither to repairing the damaged relationship nor to forward-looking action that may prevent further mistakes. A woman being treated for breast cancer tells this story about her oncologist. After their initial appointment, at which her treatment plan was discussed in detail, the oncologist faxed the woman a document that contained incorrect information about the stage of her cancer. After an agonizing delay of several days, during which the woman feared that her cancer might be far more advanced than she had been led to believe, and when her repeated calls to the oncologist were not returned, she spoke with a nurse in the oncologist's office. The nurse told the woman that the document was incorrect and that the oncologist had been aware of the mistake. She also acknowledged the woman's emotional distress and that this distress had been exacerbated by the oncologist's failure to return the repeated calls. The nurse then got the oncologist on the phone, who proceeded to offer this "apology": "I'm sorry, but I had 36 patients that day, and we mixed up your records with the other new patient's." This woman did not feel that this physician's "I'm sorry" constituted anything close to an apology for the considerable anguish his mistake, and subsequent failure to disclose the mistake, had caused her, nor did she feel that this statement conveyed any sense of accountability to her, the other patient, or the prevention of future mistakes of this kind. Although there was no medical harm resulting from this error, there was emotional harm, and also harm to the physician-patient relationship: It became impossible for this patient to trust this physician. Legal scholar Carl D. Schneider writes that a genuine apology "is offered *without defense.*"[38] In this case, the attempt to justify the mistake — I'm so busy helping all you sick people, of course I got confused when I did the paperwork, of course I couldn't return your calls, what do you expect? — turns the so-called apology into an insult, in much the same way as the failure to apologize translates into an insult.

The Colorado and Oregon "I'm sorry" laws, and the other examples of this trend, are part of the larger political trend movement toward tort reform, which is generally understood by physicians as laws and policies aimed at curbing malpractice lawsuits. The "I'm sorry" laws may be supported by consumer groups and by advocates of mediation as an alternative means of dispute resolution. By lessening if not eliminating the legal risk attached to expressions of sympathy and fault, these laws may eventually contribute to changing the way physicians approach the aftermath of medical mistakes. However, it is important to ask, what do these laws do for injured patients? Not a lot. At best, some of these laws may encourage hospitals to reconsider the way they — that is to say, their lawyers and risk managers — advise physicians concerning the legal ramifications of disclosing their mistakes to patients and offering apologies that convey an acknowledgment of the patient's suffering and of the physician's responsibility for the mistake that caused the suffering. Yet some health care systems and malpractice insurers have been giving physicians essentially the same advice for years, relying on ethical norms concerning truth telling and cultural expectations concerning apology, rather than on the protection of a statute. Several of the health care systems that are the most deeply committed to disclosure and apology after mistakes also offer compensation to injured patients as part of their disclosure policy and practices, but the "I'm sorry" laws themselves make no provision for compensating patients for their injuries. They are designed to protect physicians, not patients, and yet, perversely, they may leave physicians and hospitals exposed around the issue of compensation. Commenting on this paradox in the larger tort-reform trend, Lucian Leape, the preeminent expert on medical error in the United States, concludes: "Unless we have a fair compensation scheme — which we should because it's the right thing to do — people will still have an incentive to sue."[39]

Simply protecting a statement that includes the words "I'm sorry," and that may even include an admission of fault — "I'm sorry that I made a mistake that injured you" — may encourage such statements, but is not sufficient to protect the interests of the injured patient. These words alone do not materially change the patient's circumstances or ensure that the patient will be dealt with fairly in other respects. An apology, whether "safe" or "unsafe" under the law, is a responsible first action, but it is not the only action that a physician or hospital ought to take to make justice for patients and families after medical mistakes. It is intriguing that Lee Taft, who rightly criticizes mediators and others who characterize apologies as magic words that fend off lawsuits, characterizes apology as a "performative utterance," a phrase used by cultural anthropologists to describe words that make something happen. The Miranda warning and "I now pronounce you husband and wife" are everyday examples of performative utterances. Failure to "Mirandize" a suspect may cause a judge to throw out a case, and a couple knows they are married only when they hear "I now pronounce you . . ." Certainly, the words "I'm sorry" are frequently discussed as though they have the transformative power of these phrases, as though they alone have the power to "heal" an injured patient. And offering an apology is an action, just as disclosing a mistake is an action. But *apology*, the actions that acknowledge harm, responsibility, and regret, and *repentance*, the actions that materially restore the injured person to health, that repair the relational breach, and that safeguard against future injuries, are not at all the same thing. Bishop Desmond Tutu makes this distinction between the two types of actions: "If you take my pen and say you are sorry, but don't give me the pen back, nothing has happened."[40] If a physician apologizes to an injured patient, if a physician genuinely feels remorse for having injured the patient, if a physician acknowledges that the mistake was her fault, but there are no provisions for fairly compensating the patient for the cost of medical care and lost wages resulting from the injury and no provisions for helping this physician to avoid injuring other patients, nothing has happened.[41]

Therefore, the "I'm sorry" law trend may be encouraging in some respects, but it is an incomplete remedy for the problem of medical harm. Dietrich Bonhoeffer observed that "the villain and the saint" are never touched by efforts to systematize ethics, as saints and villains are transgressors by definition.[42] Some people will always do the right thing, and some will always do the wrong thing, regardless of whether there is a law or a code of ethics to spell out what is permitted and what is not permitted and regardless of whether the principles underlying these guides to practice promote or sabotage justice. Commenting on the particular folly of assuming that what is legal is synonymous with what is right, Martin Luther King, Jr., used an example from Bonhoeffer's own era. "We can never forget," King wrote while jailed on a civil disobedience charge, "that everything Hitler did in Germany was 'legal.' "[43]

With King's eloquent caution in mind, we may still ask how likely the "I'm sorry" laws are to encourage the practice of apology as part of the disclosure of medical harm and the care of injured patients and their families. The fact that patient safety advocates in Colorado supported that state's law suggests that some patients and families, and those who work with them, view the legal protection of apology as a measure that will enhance the care of patients and families after medical harm by allowing the words "I'm sorry" to be part of this care, rather than words to be avoided at all costs. But merely protecting apologies is not the same as encouraging them. Genuine apologies are never fun to make. They are humbling, and who among us, least of all a highly trained physician who made a mistake while trying to make things better, likes to be humbled? Yet regardless of the precise legal status of the words "I'm sorry" in any particular state at any particular moment, apologizing to a patient after harming that patient is always the right thing to do for that patient, at that particular moment, in the aftermath of harm. Patients who are harmed should receive apologies that acknowledge and take responsibility for the harm. Physicians should not be afraid to make such apologies, and institutions should actively support physicians in the difficult, humbling, necessary practice of apology after harm. And apology after medical harm is rarely, if ever, the only right thing to do: If physicians and hospitals want to say they're sorry, they must also find ways to give the pen back.

CHAPTER SIX

Repentance

Apology and compensation are intimately linked as ethical responses to harm, despite efforts, sometimes well intentioned, sometimes calculated, to separate them. Legal scholar Jonathan Cohen, writing about the status of apology under the law, concludes that "decoupling" apology from liability — that is, finding ways to allow responsible parties to apologize to those whom they have harmed without putting themselves in legal jeopardy — is, for the most part, a good idea, as long as responsible parties are willing to have a "different conversation" with those whom they have harmed around the issue of liability and fair compensation.[1] Yet Cohen also argues that a responsible party may, in good conscience, make a *sincere* apology as a strategic effort to ward off a lawsuit, although he acknowledges that there are problems with this position. If a sincere apology is so legalistically constructed as to be meaningless to the harmed party, it may not have the desired effect, whereas proposing apology as a legal strategy — say "I'm sorry" and maybe they won't sue you — may encourage unethical sham apologies.[2]

Other commentators, including proponents of alternative dispute resolution (ADR) methods such as mediation, have pointed out that overemphasizing the "magic" of apology in resolving disputes without litigation can act against the interests of harmed parties if apology alone, and not apology *and* fair compensation — saying you're sorry *and* giving the pen back — is presented, implied, or inferred as the appropriate goal of mediation. An important study that compared outcomes of ADR by gender and ethnicity and documented patterns of lower monetary settlements to those participants who wielded the least social and economic power suggests that unequal power relationships in the larger society may measurably influence "neutral" dispute-resolution processes.[3] Feminist critics, including some who are mediators themselves and who generally support ADR, suggest that there may be unintended hazards for women in dispute-resolution processes that seem to privilege communication over compensation, rather than integrating the issue of fair compensation into honest and respectful communication.[4] "Decoupling" apology from compensation, or presenting apology as equivalent to or more valuable than compensation, may work against the interests of injured parties, by failing to guarantee that a "different conversation" about compensation will in fact ever take place, or by suggesting in various ways that there is something unseemly about even putting the issue of compensation — of *money* — on the table.

The tort system is a terrible way to compensate injured patients. As long as compensation is available only if the three-part legal test for negligence can be satisfied, the majority of medical injuries will remain uncompensated, because most medical injuries are not the result of negligence but occur within the standard of care. So long as malpractice awards are tied to lost wages, low-income patients and their families will have difficulty even finding a lawyer willing to take their cases, regardless of the severity of the harm. Similarly, if the harm suffered is less severe and the potential monetary stakes are lower, lawyers will not find it worth their time to take the case. Even when a patient or family wins a malpractice award, it may be reduced on appeal, and it may be years between the injury and the final resolution of the case, with attorneys' fees and other litigation costs further reducing the amount actually awarded to the patient or family.

The damage inflicted on the relationship between the patient-as-litigant and the physician-as-defendant also argues against the tort system as a remedy for most medical harms. Being sued is a deeply traumatic experience for the individual physicians who are the targets of malpractice suits. Physicians who have been sued, and even those who have not been sued but have witnessed among their peers the brutal psychological, professional, and often financial impact of defending malpractice suits, may become suspicious of patients in general, equivocal or cynical about their professional obligation to disclose mistakes, and prone to conflating "nuisance" or "frivolous" lawsuits with cases in which a patient was seriously harmed as the result of a mistake. On-the-record comments by physicians to the effect that "malpractice is just an opportunity for some people to make some easy money"[5] and that injured patients who sued their doctors were trying to "turn bad luck into good luck"[6] suggest the extent to which fear of being sued, mistrust of the tort system, and attendant demonization of personal-injury lawyers and their clients may render physicians unable, or unwilling, to acknowledge the impact of mistakes on patients and families, as opposed to the impact of mistakes on physicians themselves.

Yet to say that the tort system does a bad job of compensating injured patients and has a negative effect on physician-patient relations is not to say that it is impossible to fairly compensate these patients. As surgeon and patient-safety pioneer Lucian Leape observes, as long as there is no system in place to deliver fair compensation, as long as the tort system remains the sole venue for many patients and families to attempt to secure compensation for medical injuries, there will be lawsuits.[7] Therefore, physicians, hospital administrators, and others who are in favor of tort reform ought to commit themselves to ensuring that all injured patients are fairly compensated for the physical and financial consequences of medical mistakes, rather than merely working to limit the awards that a very few patients might receive through the all-or-nothing tort system or by vilifying patients who do attempt to win compensation through lawsuits. This chapter will examine three fair-compensation programs currently operating in different regions of the United States, paying particular attention to how these programs are integrated into the practices of disclosure and apology, of saying "I'm sorry" *and* giving the pen back.

First, a few words about that awfully religious-sounding word in the title of this chapter, that middle, often overlooked, step between apology and forgiveness: repentance. In discussions of systems approaches to the problem of medical harm and the care of injured patients and families, the word "accountability" fulfills something of a similar function, in that, like "repentance," it describes the concrete, real-time responsibilities of the responsible party toward the harmed party. Virginia A. Sharpe, a philosopher and clinical ethicist who has studied the problem of medical harm for many years, describes the need for a shift in thinking about accountability, from "backward-looking" accountability, which too frequently is reduced to blaming and shaming an individual for screwing up, to "forward-looking" accountability, which acknowledges both the mistake and the harm resulting from the mistake, but moves forward to address the system's responses to the mistake and the harm.[8] Fair compensation, the subject of this chapter, is not synonymous with the larger issue of accountability, which also encompasses activities such as error-prevention and error-reduction efforts, error reporting, quality improvement, and all aspects of disclosure. But fair compensation, because it is so concrete — giving the pen back — and because it requires engagement with the injured party, is a good way to understand and to critique calls for systems accountability. Looking ahead is important; indeed, it's the only way to prevent errors. And limiting accountability to looking backward, so that a "responsible" (i.e., guilty) individual can be "held accountable" (i.e., blamed), cannot improve the system as a whole, because it reinforces the myth that all mistakes can be attributed solely to "bad apples." But forward-looking accountability must not be misconstrued as an activity that focuses only on the future, or on abstract goals, at the expense of the present-day needs of the patients and families — and clinicians — affected by past medical mistakes. Nor should it be reduced to the "let's have closure and move on" mantra heard so often in our culture following trauma or scandal. With respect to fairly compensating injured patients, the case studies in this chapter clarify that justice demands that physicians and institutions go backward, not to blame and shame, but to determine what *this* patient and *this* family need, today and going forward, as the result of what happened to *them*. The goal of improving conditions for hypothetical patients and families in the future must never overlook the need for real-time repentance toward real injured patients and their families.

To understand how fair compensation, particularly when integrated into the practices of disclosure and apology, constitutes repentance after harm, it is useful to appreciate the distinction between restitution and reparations. Restitution means restoration of the actual thing — land, money, artifacts, bones, rights — that was taken from a person or a community. Reparations, by contrast, are offered when the actual thing that was lost cannot be restored. Reparations, therefore, are always symbolic on some level, a repair of damage rather than a literal return of goods.[9] Recalling Bishop Tutu's analogy, "giving the pen back" may describe an act of reparation if the original pen was destroyed and what is given back is something different, but nevertheless acceptable to the person who suffered the original loss.

Compensation after medical harm is a form of reparation in at least two senses. Fair compensation, offered as part of a health care system's formal disclosure process rather than through the tort system, symbolizes a willingness to repair the damaged relationship between injured patients and providers. It also represents a willingness to acknowledge and repair the actual damage done to the body and life of an injured patient as the result of a medical mistake. Legal scholar Martha Minow, who has studied the role of reparations in the resolution of political conflicts, concludes that reparations, in their concreteness, are so important symbolically that they may satisfy the injured party's need for apology even if the offender offering reparations never actually says the words "I'm sorry."[10] However, she argues, the reverse is not the case: A verbal apology alone cannot symbolize the action, the tangible weight, of reparations.[11] This is an important point, as commentators on apology may, in their assessment of and even enthusiasm for what one terms its "thaumaturgical"[12]—miracle-working—effect on damaged relationships, may overstate the extent to which an apology alone constitutes compensation after harm.[13] Although this may be the case in ordinary interpersonal relations, some harms are indeed quantifiable, and fair compensation may indeed involve buying someone a new pen if you can't return the old one. Minow is also skeptical of the symbolic value of apologies that are offered on behalf of the responsible party when such "official" apologies do not include compensation: "If unaccompanied by direct and immediate action, such as monetary reparations, official apologies risk seeming meaningless."[14]

In Jewish and Christian traditions, apology and repentance are part of the same process. Secular Western culture has absorbed this process so thoroughly that cultural norms such as "say you're sorry" and "do the right thing" are drummed into young children without requiring any reference to religious doctrine or practice. Nonreligious persons value the words of apology, backed up by the actions of repentance, as much as religious persons do, and may be equally offended when these words and actions are not forthcoming after harm. The importance of these cultural norms suggests that, to honor the view from below, the perspective of the injured patient, fair compensation needs to be part of the same conversation as disclosure and apology. Although disclosure is about telling the truth, it isn't *only* about telling the truth. Disclosure is also about determining the impact of medical mistakes on the lives of patients and their families and acknowledging that some injured patients have legitimate needs for compensation. Finally, providing fair compensation, together with disclosure and apology, may prevent lawsuits, because these words and actions, offered together, satisfy each of the needs—to know what happened, to have one's suffering taken se-

riously, to repair, literally and symbolically, the damage caused by the mistake —
that along with anger at nondisclosure, lack of apology, and lack of compensation, drive lawsuits.[15]

Only a handful of fair-compensation programs for injured patients in the
United States have been described in journal articles or in media accounts. To
date, only one of these programs, in existence since the late 1980s, has become
well known to researchers outside of its own institution; two others, both of
which were launched in late 1990s, have chiefly been described from within their
own systems.[16] The relative lack of descriptive accounts of established compensation programs does not necessarily mean that these are the only such efforts
around. According to a 2002 survey of risk managers at 245 U.S. hospitals, 36
percent of respondents reported that their institutions had a practice of compensating injured patients financially, whereas 82 percent of respondents reported
that their institutions typically covered the cost of medical care resulting from
the injury.[17] These figures reflect compensation after a variety of harms, not only
those resulting from mistakes, and the authors of this survey caution that well
over half of all respondents indicated an unwillingness to disclose *preventable*
harms — a category that includes mistakes — even though fully 80 percent of respondents reported that their institutions had disclosure policies or were developing such policies.[18] Nevertheless, these findings suggest risk managers are
accustomed to addressing some aspects of compensation after harm — notably,
the need for medical care — even if it is unclear whether this compensation is
accompanied by full disclosure.

However, most risk managers, or other health care administrators involved in
compensation after medical mistakes, do not publish articles about these activities, perhaps because it simply does not occur to them to do so, perhaps
because institutions committed to "zero tolerance" of errors would prefer not to
have their harmful mistakes discussed in professional journals. This is unfortunate because such accounts make an enormous practical contribution to patient-
safety efforts nationwide and help to refute the myth that "no one" compensates
injured patients unless first threatened with legal action. In describing fair compensation in terms of the disclosure process and presenting it as a workable
alternative to litigation, accounts of successful or even experimental compensation programs help allay the persistent fears associated with disclosing errors to
patients and families. And in demonstrating that the legitimate financial needs
of injured patients can be met cost-effectively without litigation — not only in
"closed" systems such as the Veterans Health Administration, but in mainstream

hospitals and even by malpractice insurers—descriptive accounts help raise the bar for institutional patient-safety efforts.

Three Fair-Compensation Programs

Lexington, Kentucky, Veterans Affairs Medical Center

The best-known fair-compensation program is that of the Lexington, Kentucky, Veterans Affairs Medical Center (VAMC), whose full-disclosure policy includes helping injured patients or their families file compensation claims without first initiating litigation.[19] The "Lexington Model" of "humanistic risk management" was designed in the late 1980s by physician Steve S. Kraman, the chair of the hospital's risk management committee, and Ginny M. Hamm, the hospital's in-house counsel.[20] After unsuccessfully defending several malpractice cases that resulted in large awards to plaintiffs, the hospital administrators realized that their strategy for contesting lawsuits was not working. Deciding that a better-prepared legal and risk management team was the key to protecting the institution, the hospital began a review of all incidents that might lead to litigation. The reviewers came across a case in which it was clear both that a patient had died as the result of negligence and that the patient's family had no idea of the circumstances of the death.[21] There was no risk of litigation from this unsuspecting family, but the discovery of this case constituted a moral turning point for the hospital's staff, which concluded that the family must be informed about the error, because the hospital's "role as caregiver" extended to the aftermath of harm caused by the hospital itself.[22]

In an influential 1999 article describing the Lexington Model, Kraman and Hamm characterize their institution's approach as "somewhat radical" in its insistence that all harms resulting from errors must be disclosed to patients and families and that full disclosure must go beyond simple truth telling.[23] When it is determined that a patient has been injured, Lexington VAMC administrators[24] meet with the patient (or, in the case of injury leading to death, the patient's family) to describe what happened, offer an apology, accept responsibility, discuss measures taken to prevent future errors, answer questions, and arrange for the patient to receive financial compensation or further medical treatment, as needed. According to Kraman and Hamm, hospital staff are happy to comply with this policy, because they believe it is "the right thing to do" for their patients.[25]

Although descriptions of the Lexington Model have tended to focus on its commitment to "extreme honesty," the Lexington VAMC's "Full Disclosure Handbook," which includes typical disclosure scenarios, makes it clear that, under this model, an institution "owes" injured patients compensation as well as information: "I want to tell you, on behalf of the hospital, how sorry we are that this happened. As this occurred here, we are responsible for it. The [hospital] owes you a full explanation and fair compensation. I can answer any questions you have about this incident and our attorney is here to explain compensation in more detail and to assist in the process."[26]

A press account of the Lexington Model notes that "hospital employees persuade the occasional reluctant victim to accept financial compensation."[27] Lexington's disclosure handbook explains the rationale for this practice: Patients and surviving family members who initially refuse fair compensation may feel resentful after some time has passed, particularly if the consequences of the injury include lost income to the family. This resentment, together with the financial burden of lost income, may prompt litigation. The hospital always advises injured patients and their families to hire their own lawyer to explain the compensation process and to represent them in settlement negotiations — another way of ensuring that the patient and family are satisfied that the compensation offer adequately covers the full consequences of the injury. Because the offer constitutes a "settlement" in legal terms, patients or families who accept compensation must waive their right to sue the federal government, which functions as the defendant in malpractice suits brought against facilities in the VA health care system.[28]

Far from encouraging lawsuits, the practice of promptly disclosing mistakes, apologizing, and offering fair compensation, according to Kraman and Hamm, "diminishes the anger and desire for revenge that often motivate patients' litigation."[29] It also proactively informs patients and families about harmful errors, rather than concealing them in an effort to avoid litigation, and has been the catalyst for improved error reporting and other patient-safety measures throughout the hospital; once hospital staff became accustomed to disclosing errors to patients and families, they "became more comfortable in reporting their own errors" within the system.[30]

As of 2000, Lexington was averaging $15,000 per settlement, compared with $98,000 for all VA hospitals.[31] Steve Kraman, one of the architects of the Lexington Model, is convinced that non-VA hospitals would see similar results, "If everybody did this nationwide, every patient who was injured would get fair compensation, the lawyers would get nothing, and you wouldn't see $12 million verdicts."[32]

Catholic Healthcare West

Because the VA health care system is a closed system — serving a limited patient population, employing its own physicians (who, as federal employees, are immune from personal liability), and able to take advantage of a Federal program to pay out compensation settlements — physicians and health care administrators who work outside this system sometimes react to the Lexington Model with skepticism, saying, "Well, that's the VA — we can't do that in *my* hospital." Yet at least one very large health care system beyond the VA has adopted a disclosure policy that is similar to the Lexington Model in its proactive approach to fair compensation after harm. Catholic Healthcare West (CHW), a San Francisco–based network of forty-one hospitals in California, Arizona, and Nevada, is the largest nonprofit health care system in the western United States.[33] Created in the mid-1980s through the affiliation of a dozen hospitals owned by two Roman Catholic religious orders, CHW has become more secular as it has grown; the system now includes several nonprofit hospitals that are neither Catholic nor religious. Even as its living link with its founding religious communities diminishes, CHW has chosen to identify with its religiously grounded core values in crafting an approach to patient safety and to interpret those values in terms of the system's present-day responsibilities to injured patients and their families.

In the late 1990s, after a series of incidents in which the system's handling of medical error was in conflict with its stated values, three senior CHW administrators (Rebecca Havlisch, the system's chief risk manager; Robert Johnson, the system's in-house counsel; and Carol Bayley, the clinical ethicist in charge of ethics and justice education throughout the CHW system) collectively identified a need to articulate what the system's core values — dignity, collaboration, justice, stewardship, and excellence — meant in everyday practice in the aftermath of medical mistakes.[34] In an article on the evolution of CHW's values-based approach to patient safety, Bayley, a philosopher by training, drew this parallel between everyday institutional expectations related to clinical and moral behavior: Just as it is not acceptable for conditions during surgery to "often" be sterile, so it should not be acceptable for an institution's practices to "often" reflect its values.[35] In response to this need, Havlisch, Johnson, and Bayley created the "Mistakes Project"; its title underscores the importance of recognizing that systems, and the people in them, are fallible, even as the project itself sought to deal more justly with all persons harmed or otherwise affected by medical mistakes.

An astute observer of institutional hierarchy, Bayley writes that "real cultural change must be a top-down effort that is met by bottom-up initiatives."[36] That is, before discrete practices that directly affected the way injured patients were treated could be put into place, CHW's religious and secular leaders first had to signal their approval, in this case by authorizing Bayley and her colleagues to draft a "philosophy of mistake management" for the CHW system. Even the phrase "mistake management" suggested that a paradigm shift from the norms of the more familiar phrase "risk management," in which the injured patient was viewed as the institution's adversary, was under way.

CHW's "Philosophy of Mistake Management" describes in detail what each of the system's core values means in practice following a mistake in which a patient is harmed. As in the Lexington Model, the issue of fair compensation is addressed as part of the disclosure of the mistake. At CHW, the obligation to tell the truth and the obligation to provide fair compensation both reflect the core value of "dignity": "Respect for a person's dignity means that we are honest and direct in communicating to a person who may have been harmed while under our care. Together with the physician, we must promptly supply all information to a person that is rightfully his or hers, including his/her medical record, the circumstances which resulted in the harm, the extent of the damages, and the right to fair compensation. Respect for the dignity of the person and good faith claims management compels us to advise an injured party about his/her right to obtain advi[c]e from legal counsel."[37]

Fair compensation is also discussed in terms of other core values. Concerning the core value of "justice," CHW's philosophy of mistake management affirms that "with physicians and other partners, justice requires that we take our fair share of the burden of a claim and expect the same of our partners."[38] Unlike the VA system, but like the majority of hospitals in the United States, CHW has had to factor its "voluntary medical staff" — physicians who are not employed directly by the hospital in which they treat patients — into its disclosure policies and practices. Providing fair compensation to injured patients has meant negotiating with physicians' malpractice insurers as well as with the system's own insurers, and dealing with the resistance of voluntary medical staff to participating in disclosure activities that might affect their own malpractice premiums following a settlement. (When CHW administrators introduced the philosophy of mistake management to their own malpractice insurers, most of the insurers said that, contrary to myth, they also advised physicians to disclose mistakes fully and promptly, to apologize, and to quickly settle cases in which a mistake resulted in harm.[39]) Compensation is also addressed in terms of the core value of "stewardship":

> From a risk management standpoint, it is axiomatic that patients are far more likely to seek legal representation if they believe that information has been concealed from them. Hence, timely disclosure of mistakes is cost effective.
>
> . . . we fairly compensate an injured party even when that involves the expenditure of CHW funds. At the same time, we are careful to share the burden of claims and suits fairly with those institutions and individuals that bear some responsibility for them. Faithfulness to the value of stewardship compels us to explore every avenue for a just settlement.[40]

After the drafting of the "Philosophy of Mistake Management," the cocreators of the Mistakes Project began meeting with professional groups throughout the huge CHW system to introduce them to this new approach to medical mistakes. In general, staff members were supportive, and one person echoed the Lexington VAMC staff in concluding that "being honest and apologizing seem naturally to be the right thing to do; lying about a mistake is learned."[41] Of course, "being honest and apologizing" are learned behaviors too.[42] They seem "natural" because of their deep cultural roots, because so many people are taught from earliest childhood that telling the truth is right, that covering up the truth is wrong, and that there are morally appropriate and inappropriate words and actions after one person has harmed another person. As such, it is not surprising that staff at both the Lexington VAMC and at CHW were more comfortable upholding policies and practices that promoted truth telling, apology, and compensation than they had been with policies and practices that did not encourage, or even suppressed, these words and actions. It feels "natural" to be in sync with cultural norms and expectations, and it feels unnatural to pretend that these norms and expectations — tell the truth, say you're sorry, do the right thing — apply everywhere *except* in clinical medicine.

One of the first groups in the CHW system introduced to the philosophy of mistake management was the risk managers, whose jobs would be most directly affected by putting the philosophy into practice. After years of educating and observing risk managers, Carol Bayley concludes that the most effective ones initiate the discussion of fair compensation by asking injured patients and their families, "What do you need, based on what happened?"[43] This question is clearly grounded in the obligation to tell patients and families the truth about "what happened," but it also serves a strategic function, by encouraging patients and families to focus on concrete needs resulting from the injury—medical expenses, lost wages, reduced income due to disability—rather than on a dollar amount. One family affected by a harmful mistake thought about this question and determined that what they really needed, based on what had happened, was a mobile home. CHW agreed that this was fair compensation, and the family got it.

COPIC

COPIC, a Denver-based insurer that provides malpractice insurance to six thousand physicians in Colorado and Nebraska, and also insures hospitals and health plans, offers another innovative fair-compensation program.[44] (COPIC was one of the sponsors of the "I'm sorry" law in Colorado, discussed in chapter 5.) The values and goals underlying COPIC's compensation program are perhaps more explicitly concerned with limiting liability and heading off costly litigation than are the approaches of the Lexington VAMC and CHW, although those institutions are also motivated by the desire to avoid litigation and are eager to demonstrate the cost-effectiveness of their strategies when compared with the cost of defending lawsuits. And whereas CHW and the Lexington VAMC integrate compensation into the disclosure policies and practices of their respective health care systems, COPIC's program operates independently of any single health care system's processes. However, the program is premised on physicians' willingness to report mistakes to COPIC and then, together with a COPIC risk manager, to disclose mistakes to patients. The company also "urge[s]" the physicians it insures to take an active role in developing disclosure policies and procedures at the hospitals in which they work.[45] In its own in-house guidelines on disclosure, COPIC advises its physicians that any unanticipated outcomes that "have a significant impact on a patient's prognosis, choices, or quality and functional ability of life"[46] should always be disclosed; the reasoning here is that if a patient suspects or finds out that such information was withheld, the likelihood of productive communication decreases while the likelihood of legal action increases.

COPIC's program is called "3Rs," which stands for "Recognize, Respond to and Resolve Patient Injury."[47] The pilot program was announced in mid-1999 and launched in October 2000.[48] Although COPIC initially sought to recruit 500 participants—300 surgeons, 200 nonsurgeons—for the project, by the end of 2003 more than 1,300 physicians were participating.[49] The stated goal of the 3Rs program at the time of its announcement and initial recruitment efforts was to improve physicians' ability to communicate with and address the needs of patients in the immediate aftermath of a mistake or other injury, "'before the physician/patient relationship is irretrievably damaged and before it escalates to a claim.'"[50] The program's core elements include a commitment to responding to injured patients within 72 hours after a physician reports an injury to COPIC's risk managers, "humanistic and effective"[51] communications; financial reimbursement for lost income and nonreimbursable medical expenses resulting from the injury, and arranging for medical care or other services that the patient may need. Payments under the 3Rs program, which is not designed to provide compensation for injuries resulting in death or for wrong-site surgeries and other major errors that continue to be handled as traditional malpractice claims, are capped at $30,000, including a maximum of $25,000 toward out-of-pocket medical expenses and a maximum of $5,000, or 50 days, of compensation for lost wages.[52] As of December 31, 2003, financial payments under the 3Rs program averaged $1,820, compared with an average of $78,741 for costs associated with investigating traditional malpractice claims even when *no* payment was made to a patient.[53]

A significant difference between COPIC's approach to compensation and the approaches of the Lexington VAMC and Catholic Healthcare West is that patients who participate in the 3Rs program cannot be represented by or otherwise make use of legal counsel during the period when compensation is being discussed, although they do not waive their right to sue and may subsequently retain counsel and pursue a formal malpractice claim if they are dissatisfied with the resolution of their case.[54] Although the difference between these two approaches to some extent turns on the distinction between a "settlement" and a "payment" after medical harm and may also reflect the more limited scale of the harms that the 3Rs program is equipped to handle, it also highlights the current reality that all fair-compensation programs are played out within the context of reducing malpractice risk and institutional exposure, resulting in a trade-off between the risk of allowing patients to seek legal counsel during negotiations over compensation and the risk of allowing patients to retain their right to sue in the future.

The difference between "settlements" versus "payments" is also germane to the issue of physicians' incentives to support and participate in efforts to integrate disclosure and compensation, and to the overall question of accountability. Whereas settlements are paid out of the responsible parties' malpractice insurance and must be reported to the National Practitioner Data Bank (NPDB), payments under the 3Rs program are covered by COPIC's own funds and are therefore not required to be reported to the NPDB.[55] This provides a major incentive for physicians to participate in the 3Rs program (as does the fact that the payments, because they are not "settlements," do not trigger increases in participating physicians' premiums), though it is worth noting that the Lexington VAMC voluntarily reports its settlements to the NPDB in the interest of accountability, even though, as a federal institution, it is not required to do so.[56] Thus, another trade-off is revealed, in this case between increasing access for individual patients to disclosure and compensation after medical harm by maximizing incentives for physicians to participate in disclosure and compensation programs, and upholding the obligation to report all settlements, including those that do not involve negligence, in the interest of transparency and patient safety nationwide.[57] A partial resolution to this dilemma is suggested by a related practice at the Lexington VAMC, which, in the interest of encouraging physicians to trust that they will be treated fairly during the disclosure process, no longer settles nuisance suits. As Steve Kraman writes, although it is "tempting" for hospitals to respond to allegations of malpractice in cases where no standard of care was breached by offering a "modest" settlement that would be less than the cost of litigating a case that a hospital expects to win, such settlements, because they must be reported to the NPDB along with the name of the physician involved in the case, work against efforts to encourage physicians to disclose actual mistakes.[58] By contrast, in refusing to settle nuisance suits, even at the risk of incurring litigation costs, the hospital signals to physicians that it takes their interests seriously, "rather than appear[ing] to be willing to sacrifice our clinician[s'] reputations to save a few thousand dollars."[59] Such a stance may, over time, and if adopted by sufficient numbers of institutions, also help to dispel the persistent and damaging image of the injured patient as greedy litigant.

An underlying principle — one may even term it a core value — of the 3Rs program is that patients' expectations matter, and patients do not expect to be injured by their physicians. As one COPIC publication on disclosure states, "it is the patient's perspective and their underlying expectation that determines if an adverse outcome is unanticipated."[60] The focus of the program is on recognizing, responding to, and resolving cases of patient *injury*, not physician *error*. Indeed, COPIC cautions physicians that a legalistic approach to selectively disclosing mistakes — as was evident in the national survey of risk managers described earlier — offers scant protection against litigation if the patient finds out or suspects that a known error that resulted in an injury was concealed, rather than being acknowledged and compensated.[61] COPIC also alerts physicians to the importance of apology as a cultural norm, stating without qualification that "patients expect apologies" after mistakes, and that "there is a difference between an apology and expressing 'being sorry about the outcome.' "[62] Reflecting on legal scholar Lee Taft's disdain for such stilted pseudoapologies as " 'I'm sorry you are suffering' "[63] — discussed in chapter 5 — it is intriguing that a malpractice insurer echoes Taft's dismissal of this scripted language, not because the pseudoapology will fail to, in Taft's opinion, "restore the moral balance" between erring physician and injured patient, but simply because the patient's expectation of appropriate behavior after harm will not be met, thereby creating a barrier to resolution and increasing the risk of litigation.

In its focus on meeting a patient's needs and expectations concerning an injury and on the active role that a physician, as opposed to an institution, must take throughout the disclosure and compensation process — given that it is the physician's insurer who is the source of compensation funds — the 3Rs program shares some similarities with a no-fault system of compensation, such as exists in the health care systems of Denmark, Finland, Sweden, and New Zealand, and, in a very limited way, in several public-sector initiatives in the United States.[64] In no-fault systems, patients who are injured as the result of avoidable mistakes in the course of appropriate treatment receive compensation for the medical or financial burden of the injury; unlike in a tort system, there is no need to satisfy a legal definition of negligence or to hold a health care provider personally liable. In a 2001 *JAMA* article assessing the potential for no-fault compensation systems to enhance error-prevention efforts in the United States by diminishing physicians' persistent fear that reporting mistakes will trigger lawsuits, authors David M. Studdert and Troyen A. Brennan of Harvard University describe how, under the Swedish no-fault system, physicians seem to perceive helping injured patients obtain compensation as "a natural extension of their therapeutic responsibility to safeguard patients' best interests." They are "actively involved" in the resolution of the majority of cases, "alerting patients to the possibility that a medical injury has occurred, referring the patient to a social worker for assistance, even helping patients to lodge claims."[65] Studdert and Brennan acknowledge that, because of the underlying structure of the health care system, the resistance of plaintiffs' attorneys to a shift away from the malpractice model, and other factors, the United States is very far from adopting a no-fault model nationally. However, they argue that no-fault programs that offer "speedy, equitable, affordable, and predictable" compensation to injured patients while addressing other patient-safety goals, including reporting, disclosure, and quality improvement, can and ought to be tried at the state level.⁶⁶ It would seem that such an experiment, in practice if not in name, is indeed underway in Colorado, and that participating physicians who were initially skeptical of the 3Rs program, fearing that discussing mistakes and addressing compensation with injured patients would trigger malpractice claims, are willing to support a radically different approach to thinking about and resolving the needs of injured patients. In one case cited in the COPIC literature, a surgeon who reported an incident in which he perforated a patient's bowel during a laparoscopy, which resulted in the need for hospitalization, further surgery, parenteral nutrition, and home care, expressed satisfaction with the support he received from the 3Rs risk manager, who coached him for the meeting with the patient, at which he disclosed the mistake and its ensuing complications. The patient, moreover, was described as expressing "great satisfaction with the speed and ease of obtaining benefits under the program."⁶⁷

Most people can recite some version of the Golden Rule, which, with reference to Christian teachings, is often expressed as "do unto others as you would have them do unto you,"⁶⁸ although many versions of this ethical principle exist within other cultures and religious traditions. COPIC's guidance to physicians on disclosing medical mistakes concludes with this version of the rule: "we must treat our patients as we would want ourselves or our families to be treated."⁶⁹ Or as COPIC's CEO, Jerome Buckley, M.D., explained in an interview, "You can fan the flames of the problem by not being there and communicating. Or you can say, 'I'm sorry this happened . . . and I'll be there to help you.' "⁷⁰

Conclusion

Christian ethicist Larry L. Rasmussen, referring to the work of communitarian theorist Philip Selznick, identifies the marks of a morally healthy community as "historicity, identity, mutuality, plurality, autonomy, participation, and integration."⁷¹ Although Rasmussen is principally concerned with analyzing the role of religious institutions as loci for moral community within civil society, these marks of moral community may apply to secular institutions, with respect to how these institutions identify, interpret, and act on their core values. Moral community can announce itself in unexpected ways. For example, the administrators of the Lexington VAMC did not set out to create a model full-disclosure policy: Their initial objective was to do a better job in preparing for and winning lawsuits. However, the readiness with which lawyers and risk managers — administrators whose jobs are defined in terms of institutional protection — recognized that the system's "role as caregiver" extended to the families that were unaware of the cause of a loved one's death suggests an underlying awareness of the hospital as moral community. This recognition, in turn, was the catalyst for the sort of "prospective" or "forward-looking" accountability that Virginia Sharpe argues is incumbent on all "who are engaged in the healing enterprise,"[72] an enterprise that by its very nature is forward looking. Thus, having acknowledged that the system's cherished role — and by extension, the role of every person within this system — as "caregiver" ought not to be vacated by the fact of a medical mistake or other bad outcome, the lawyers and risk managers began to question themselves about the specific responsibilities binding on this role after a patient suffers an injury while in their care.

The VA health care system exists to serve veterans, who have earned the right to lifetime medical care. Most of its patients are elderly, poor, and vulnerable, often dependent on their local VA hospital for long-term care, during which time they would become well known to hospital staff. The norms of moral community, in particular, historicity, identity, and autonomy, were sufficiently embedded within the culture of the Lexington VAMC to allow its administrators to recognize that concealing a known error from a family that, literally, did not know enough to sue would violate the hospital's distinctive identity and historic caregiving role and the family's right to know the truth about a patient's care. This insight led to the development of policies and practices that sought to uncover errors, fully and promptly inform and fairly compensate patients, and take the risk that patients and families, once informed, offered compensation, and thereby recognized as participants in the process of full disclosure, might still sue. As a result, this system's culture was changed even as its core values were reaffirmed, and the implementation of a full-disclosure policy strengthened this moral community through concrete practices judged by all to be "the right thing to do." The discernment process at Catholic Healthcare West was similar, as administrators asked themselves how their vast and increasingly pluralistic system could interpret and practice the values, integral to its history and identity, in its care of injured patients and their families. As Carol Bayley writes concerning this process: "because [CHW's] values of dignity, collaboration, stewardship, justice and excellence are the foundational reasons the system was formed, its behavior as a system must be shaped by them or it risks forsaking its identity. 'Values' that do not affect actions are hardly worthy of the name. Disclosure was the bloom, not the root."[73]

Even at COPIC, an institution that does not itself deliver health care, and which would appear to be the farthest removed from the perspective of injured patients and most protective of physicians, administrators recognized that the patient's perspective and participation was the key, ethically and strategically, to designing a fair-compensation system, and that physicians needed to be encouraged to see themselves as patients so that they might recognize why injured patients valued honest communication and attentiveness to the impact of medical injuries on their health and lives so much.

The processes that administrators at the Lexington Veterans Administration Medical Center, Catholic Healthcare West, and COPIC describe in developing their patient-centered approaches to disclosing medical harm and providing fair compensation to injured patients, while informed by the cultures and vocabularies of these quite different institutions, can be summarized as follows: because we are part of the "healing enterprise," we are responsible for putting patients' interests first. To put patients' interests first after medical harm means to identify the real needs of real patients, not to indulge in counterproductive blaming and shaming of clinicians. To identify these real needs, we must become accustomed to talking openly and honestly with patients. We must ask them, "What do you need, based on what happened?" then listen respectfully to their responses, and work collaboratively with them to address their needs. We must support physicians in their efforts to talk openly and honestly with real patients, and in so doing, to diminish their fears and stereotypes concerning "angry" and "litigious" patients.

Repentance after harm—giving the pen back—requires direct engagement with the injured party and attentiveness to their stated needs. This negotiation, in turn, establishes the necessary conditions for forgiveness, the final, in some ways most problematic, most mythologized, and least understood part of the relational process enacted after one person harms another person. Forgiveness is the domain of the injured party, even though it is often not recognized as such. The next chapter explores the nature of forgiveness in the aftermath of medical harm.

CHAPTER SEVEN

Forgiveness

The title of the landmark Institute of Medicine report on medical error, *To Err Is Human*, is derived from Alexander Pope's "Essay on Criticism" (1711): "To err is human; to forgive, divine" (l. 525).[1] Given how familiar this proverb is in its entirety, it is striking that the IOM report itself contains no reference to forgiveness, divine or otherwise, in its treatment of medical error, even as its title hints at a fundamental relationship between error and forgiveness. A systems approach to medical error, the approach advocated by the IOM and the national patient-safety movement alike, may similarly "forget" to engage forgiveness as a tool for addressing the needs of all parties affected by medical error: patients, families, clinicians, administrators, and institutions. Insights from religion and related aspects of culture may help clinicians, ethicists, and other professionals involved in nurturing "cultures of safety" within health care institutions, or medical educators responsible for introducing students to the sensitive issue of their own fallibility and its potential impact on patients, to recognize the restorative role that forgiveness has long played between individuals and within communities and to incorporate forgiveness into ways of thinking about and addressing medical harm. What follows is a broad "religious studies" rather than a strictly "theological" or "doctrinal" perspective on forgiveness, one that incorporates insights from Jewish and Christian social ethics, ritual studies, the sociology of medicine, and medical anthropology, as well as from clinicians themselves. Dena Davis defines the task of the religious ethicist working on clinical issues as describing what real people really believe and how they really act, a definition worth keeping in mind whenever the word "religion" comes up in relation to clinical medicine.[2]

That said, several concepts borrowed from Christian theologian Dietrich Bonhoeffer—"cheap grace" among them—are integral to the argument against what might be termed forgiveness as a self-interpreting principle. What is meant by this phrase is a way of formulating "forgiveness" so that its relational character—the actions that various persons undertake in relation to one another so forgiveness can take place—is forgotten. This relational understanding of forgiveness may be replaced by a cheap grace that, in formulating forgiveness as automatic, either acknowledges no role for the injured person as agent of forgiveness, or assumes that this person should offer forgiveness in the absence of truth telling, apology, fair compensation, or other goods that we might place under the ethical principle of justice. In cases of medical harm, a cheap-grace approach on the part of professional caregivers, including clinicians, chaplains, social workers, or pastors, may also place pressure on injured patients and their families to forgive automatically—by reminding them, in subtle and not-so-subtle ways, that "good" people are "forgiving," or by assuring them that offering forgiveness will bring them "closure," or by telling them that, after all, nobody *meant* to harm them—even as these patients and their families remain profoundly distressed by not knowing what really happened, or by the absence of any acknowledgment of their suffering by those directly responsible for it.

In avoiding nonrelational approaches to forgiveness, we must keep in mind that forgiveness is a "Janus" word, in that it holds contradictory meanings—to engage and to detach—that are often conflated or insufficiently distinguished in everyday conversation and in scholarly discourse: One of the most important questions you can ask about forgiveness is what *you* mean when you use this word. In the Jewish and Christian traditions, the deepest meaning of forgiveness is *detachment*. Forgiveness as cheap grace, as entitlement rather than outcome, ignores this deep meaning by refusing to ask what those harmed through medical mistakes may need to achieve detachment, or by pressuring them into engagement or acquiescence, even into a divine, salvific role, instead of allowing detachment to take place over time—in what the Christian Bible refers to as *kairos*, the appropriate time, as opposed to *chronos*, chronological time — once justice has been secured.[3] Arguing for a definition of forgiveness after medical harm that holds detachment as the ultimate goal of the process does not mean that injured patients — or clinicians who have made errors — should simply be encouraged to "detach" from incidents of medical harm, and from their feelings concerning these incidents. Even in mundane interpersonal situations, forgiveness-as-detachment can be problematic: After we have succeeded in emotionally detaching ourselves from a painful situation, we may still hesitate to *say* "I forgive you" if we believe that, by doing so, we are excusing bad behavior rather than affirming changed behavior.

Before turning to Jewish and Christian traditions and social ethics around error and forgiveness, one final caution. Though these traditions are powerful, if not always acknowledged, influences on Western culture and Western medicine, they are not universal. Even informal conversations with clinicians and scholars knowledgeable about non-Western religious and cultural traditions and expectations can help to dispel the notion that forgiveness, in particular, is universally understood as a principle, norm, or religious or secular practice.[4] Recalling Arthur Kleinman's definition of the "category fallacy" — the "imposition of a classification scheme onto members of societies for whom it holds no validity" — is instructive.[5] It would not be appropriate to talk about the "Buddhist" or "Hindu" understanding of forgiveness, *not* because these traditions are "unforgiving," but because "forgiveness" as a metaphor for a relationship between autonomous persons simply may not work in traditions in which a concept of the self as independent from other persons or one's past lives is not the norm. For example, in traditions such as Buddhism in which suffering is recognized as an inevitable characteristic of human existence, compassion (literally, "suffering with"), not forgiveness, may be the predominant metaphor for the repair of damaged relationships. At a time when one in five physicians practicing in the United States was born and raised in Asia, as was one in four foreign-born residents of the United States, it is ever more important to be aware of the extent to which allegedly "universal" norms and rituals concerning error and forgiveness are grounded in Western culture, Western religions, and Western ideas about the self.[6] Those of us who may, on occasion, be responsible for doing religious ethics — for describing what real people really believe and how they really act — must also be aware of any tendencies on our own part to simplify, sentimentalize, or appropriate non-Western metaphors for complex ethical relationships.

Forgiveness in Jewish and Christian Social Ethics

The root word *het'* appears 595 times in the Hebrew Bible, more than four times more often than its nearest synonym.[7] This word is usually translated into English simply as "sin," but its oldest meaning—a meaning that has parallels in other ancient Near Eastern cultures—is to "miss the mark," like an archer who takes aim at a target and misses it, or a traveler who misses the correct turn.[8] *Het'* is also used to describe breaches of social ethics, as when someone "misses" an opportunity to assist another. It has a theological dimension when one misses with respect to one's relationship with God, or in the performance of religious rites.

What is interesting about *het'* is that it truly means "missing the mark"—that is, error, not necessarily "sin" in the post-Augustinian sense of original sin or moral taint—requiring close attention to context to determine whether a given error was intentional, unconscious, or avoidable, a matter of judgment, skill, experience, or character. As such, the word and its associated images may make a hermeneutical contribution to understanding how different actors know medical mistakes. The same incident of "missing the mark" may be framed as a technical error by the culture of medicine, as a risk management problem by hospital lawyers, as a moral wrong, an injustice, perhaps even a sin, by the injured patient or the patient's family, and as spiritual and psychological devastation by the individual clinicians involved. By appreciating the different ways in which a medical mistake may be interpreted, we may better comprehend how the expectations of stakeholders concerning the resolution of such cases may differ and conflict.

Within the Jewish and Christian traditions, forgiveness works roughly like this: God forgives the error itself, whereas the injured party forgives the individual who has made the error. Thus, forgiveness has both a divine and a human component and encompasses two relationships, one between a human being and God, the other between human beings. Furthermore, forgiveness is a response to two discrete actions or series of actions: an acknowledgment of the error by the person who has made it, the practice often called "confession," which is inclusive of disclosure and apology; and an effort by this person to make amends for the harm he or she has done, the practice or practices often called "repentance" or "atonement." In these traditions, therefore, forgiveness is properly understood as the outcome of a relational ethical process.

Jewish traditions concerning forgiveness emphasize human agency to a somewhat greater extent than do Christian traditions, in which divine agency, often represented by clergy, may be more prominent. For example, *kapparah*, the Hebrew word for atonement, refers to the reconciliation of the person who has committed an error with the person he or she has injured.[9] The error is forgiven only when the injured person has been sufficiently appeased, a process that may involve concrete restitution—the word *kapparah* comes from a legal term for compensation—and that is ritually enacted by observant Jews each year prior to Yom Kippur.[10] The traditional Jewish understanding of atonement as the reconciliation of *persons* thus requires the injured party, as the human agent of forgiveness, to play an active role in the repentance of the person responsible for his injury. If taken literally, this expectation may be oppressive to the injured party, who may wish neither to engage directly with this person, nor to be held to her time frame for atonement. In recent years, the Kabbalist concept of *tikkun olam*, or "repairing the world" through acts that promote social justice, has come to be associated with the traditional rituals of Yom Kippur, extending the idea of atonement beyond the reconciliation of individuals and toward communal responsibility for addressing injustice and the needs of the most vulnerable members of society.[11]

The extensive use of the Lord's Prayer in Christian worship makes it a window through which to glimpse how individual perspectives on error and forgiveness may be grounded in formative religious influences and internalized norms. The best-known version of this prayer comes from the Gospel according to Matthew and includes the phrase, "forgive us our debts, as we also have forgiven our debtors."[12] The "debt" language, which has many antecedents in the Hebrew Bible, means God forgives sin by releasing the believer from the error that is holding him captive, and that one human being forgives another by detaching from that person, and the harm that person has caused, as a source of pain, anger, and injustice. The underlying metaphor is the cancellation of a financial debt that can never be repaid; the metaphor itself is grounded in a culture in which debt-servitude was common. The shorter, probably older version of this prayer found in Luke's Gospel makes even clearer the extent to which these early Christian texts are grounded in the Jewish understanding of how forgiveness works: "forgive us our sins, for we ourselves forgive everyone indebted to us."[13] God forgives the error, but people must first forgive one another.

Christian paradigms of error and forgiveness may stress personal salvation (the repair of one's relationship with God) over the concrete making of amends to the injured party (the repair of one's relationship with another human being).

These tendencies can lead to a truncation, even a perversion, of the process of forgiveness that Bonhoeffer memorably characterizes in *Discipleship* as "cheap grace . . . cut-rate forgiveness . . . grace as doctrine, as principle, as system."[14] In this "system," disclosure, apology, and repentance — all the traditional, specific responsibilities of the person who has harmed another — are eliminated, as forgiveness is elevated to a "general truth." These are tough, even shocking words, coming from a Lutheran pastor whose tradition taught that Christians did not earn forgiveness through their own deeds, but had it freely bestowed upon them by God: As Luther himself famously wrote, "Everything is forgiven through grace."[15]

Yet what is free is not without value, and Bonhoeffer lambastes his church for treating a divine gift as though it were "bargain-basement goods": "The world finds in this church a cheap cover-up for its sins, for which it shows no remorse and from which it has even less desire to be set free."[16] Bonhoeffer's "world" is Nazi Germany, and "this church" is one that, by and large, acquiesced to evil rather than defying it, allowing itself to be used by the regime rather than working on behalf of the regime's victims. In Bonhoeffer's analysis, the Nazi-affiliated Reich church is the ultimate failed system.

Bonhoeffer's cheap-grace formulation has been used by Christian feminist ethicists to critique what Pamela Cooper-White calls "an ethic of instant forgiveness" among well-intentioned pastors and other counselors who encourage trauma survivors to forgive abusers who refuse to acknowledge or repent of their actions, and to do so even before "uncovering enough of the factual story to know what really happened."[17] It is also useful to discussions on the ethics of medical harm, in its criticism of forgiveness understood in terms of a "principle" or "system" that reflexively protects those who cause harm, even inadvertently, at the expense of those who suffer as the result of harm. When forgiveness is embraced, unexamined, as a self-evident principle — something that good people do because it's the right thing to do — rather as the outcome of a process that requires something of the one whose actions have led to harm, it may be misunderstood as a surrogate for the ethical principle of justice: The right thing to do after I have harmed you is for *you* to forgive *me*. And when discourse on medical error misuses the language of "systems" to dodge the issue of individual responsibility, or when the "factual story" about a patient's health, including injury resulting from error, is withheld from that patient, the ethical principle of respect for persons is undermined. In either case, what is ignored is what Bonhoeffer, in his *Ethics*, calls the "concrete place" of ethics — here, the reality of human suffering resulting from harm — and its attendant responsibilities.[18]

In recent years, forgiveness has captured the attention of science. A Campaign for Forgiveness Research, an initiative of the John Marks Templeton Foundation that promotes the scientific study of forgiveness, has sought to support 60 research projects on "the power of forgiveness and reconciliation" in four categories: forgiveness among individuals, among families, and among nations, and the biology and human evolution of forgiveness.[19] Although none of the projects funded to date focuses on forgiveness after medical harm, information published online by Templeton-funded researchers focusing on "forgiveness among individuals" appears to suggest that responsibility for repairing damaged interpersonal relationships lies with the person who extends or withholds forgiveness. Thus, the Heartland Forgiveness Project at the University of Kansas describes "persons who are stuck in unforgiving, unproductive patterns of interacting with themselves, other people, or situations" as those who may benefit from "forgiveness interventions."[20] The Stanford Forgiveness Project, which asserts "all major religious traditions and wisdoms extol the value of forgiveness," describes its focus as "training forgiveness to ameliorate the anger and distress involved in feeling hurt . . . the need for forgiveness emerges from a body of work demonstrating harmful effects of unmanaged anger and hostility on health," and offers its "unique and practical definition of forgiveness," which "consists primarily of taking less personal offense, reducing anger and the blaming of the offender, and developing increased understanding of situations that often lead to feeling hurt and angry."[21]

Clinical research by developmental psychologist Robert Enright and others strongly suggests that the ability to forgive is a marker of psychological health and may be indispensable to the healing of relationships.[22] However, identifying forgiveness as a norm or virtue characteristic of a physically, emotionally, and morally healthy person without closely examining the roles that disclosure, apology, and repentance play in allowing one person to forgive another potentially conflates someone who has been injured through medical harm or other trauma with someone who has a tendency to "feel hurt" and "take offense." As the sole agent of forgiveness in this scenario, the injured person must both be good *and* be God, responsible for saving herself and other people from her own unhealthy, "unproductive" anger.

Forgiveness Rituals in Western Medical Culture

Forgiveness after medical mistakes — of certain persons, by certain persons — is built into the culture of Western medicine. Charles L. Bosk's classic sociological study, *Forgive and Remember: Managing Medical Failure*, provides detailed and by all accounts still-relevant descriptions of forgiveness norms and practices among surgeons.[23] Bosk reports that among his subjects, the practice of forgiving errors "operates as a deterrence" to future errors, as the "subordinate" who is forgiven by his or her superior "becomes more vigilant" in patient care and more likely to ask for help when confronted by complications (178). And because what these surgeons describe as the " 'hair-shirt' ritual" of "self-criticism, confession, and forgiveness" is enacted before one's peers during the Mortality and Morbidity Conference, the ritual "also serves to reintegrate offenders into the group" and reaffirm group norms: "Since in time all make errors in techniques, all are obliged in time to go before the group and humble themselves. Through this practice of confession and forgiveness, the group exacts the allegiance of all its members to its standards" (178–79).

Bosk's richly descriptive account of the hair-shirt ritual of M&M as practiced by surgeons allows readers to identify vestiges of ancient Jewish and Christian practices concerning forgiveness.[24] Both Jewish and Christian communities have long incorporated ritualized confession into their most solemn rites, most notably on Yom Kippur in the Jewish tradition and on Ash Wednesday in the Roman Catholic and other Christian traditions; Bosk notes that such practices are common in monasteries (178). The "hair-shirt" that functions here as a metaphor for "self-criticism" was (and is) a real garment, woven of animal hair and worn as an act of penance during religious rites and as an ascetic practice.[25] We can even see, in the sequencing of ritual actions — confession, forgiveness, and then repentance through professional vigilance — a parallel with the reordering of Christian penitential rites in the late medieval period, as the practice of individual confession, followed by absolution and then by the performance of penitential acts assigned by one's parish priest, took hold.[26] Viewed through the lens of Western religious tradition, the M&M hair-shirt ritual and related penitential practices are neither modern nor wholly secular, whether contemporary participants recognize the ancient cultural roots of their professional ritual.

What is perhaps most striking in Bosk's account is the part played by the erring surgeon's superior, who combines religious and secular roles, functioning as deity, high priest, judge, pastor, peer group representative, and injured party, forgiving both the error itself and the person who makes the error. According to a taxonomy devised by moral philosopher J. L. Austin, who catalogued the ways rituals can fail to fulfill their cultural, religious, or psychological functions through "infelicitous performances," this conflation of roles constitutes a "ritual misapplication": a legitimate ceremony that fails because of the involvement of inappropriate persons.[27] The hair-shirt ritual, *qua* ritual, fails because it excludes the patient, whose roles as injured party and as human agent of forgiveness are usurped by the erring surgeon's superior. (The surgeons who participate in this ritual do not perceive this failure, because they would not expect patients to be part of their community and its professional rites.[28]) The patient has no role, no voice, and no representation within this private ritual and cannot rely on it for justice and for the possibility of being able to forgive and to heal. This is *not* to say that injured patients should be included in M&M. It is to say that the ritual of confession, repentance, and forgiveness may be as culturally important to patients as it is already understood to be among physicians, and it should be available to them in an appropriate venue.

The hair-shirt ritual may be infelicitous in another way. When clinicians and hospital chaplains talk about the topic of forgiveness after medical error, *self-forgiveness* emerges as a constant theme. Members of both of these professions stressed that some form of self-forgiveness was essential in restoring confidence and morale after incidents of medical harm, even as one physician acknowledged that although self-forgiveness is "something we all have to face when we make an error that harms someone . . . It is hard to get physicians to think in these terms."[29] Clinicians do not tend to characterize existing institutional processes, such as M&M, as capable, in and of itself, of helping those who have made errors to forgive themselves. Instead, the ability to have private, unguarded conversations with colleagues (what one physician called a "cadre of friends") or chaplains (described as a "safe space") in which they could discuss incidents of medical error and their own roles in and emotions concerning these incidents, appeared to be the single most important factor in the clinicians' ability to forgive themselves.[30]

One physician questioned the appropriateness of the term "self-forgiveness" and the theological premise underlying it: that one could be the agent of one's own salvation. Taken literally, self-forgiveness would be another example of cheap grace, in which the other — the injured party, God — is pushed out of the frame, whereas the person who has made the error is forgiven without any assurance that the relational actions traditionally described as confession and repentance have taken or will take place. This physician suggested an alternative definition for so-called self-forgiveness — "freedom from guilt and self-hatred" — while arguing that forgiveness itself must be understood to be relational: "there must be a self-transcending aspect to forgiveness — or it does not occur."[31]

Among clinicians, the need for self-forgiveness was held in tension with the belief that there was not "much of a possibility" of being forgiven by a patient or a patient's family after medical harm.[32] There is in these words a poignant echo of Christopher Marlowe's version of the Faust legend: In his despair, Dr. Faustus believes—incorrectly—that his "offense can never be pardoned" (*Dr. Faustus* [1604], Scene 14). Lest the contemporary reader imagine spiritual despair to be a quaintly "religious" notion or literary conceit, here are some of the words that clinicians used to describe their responses to their own mistakes: "devastated"; "heartsick . . . demoralized, worthless."[33] These clinicians also reported that even peripheral involvement in an error—referring a patient for a procedure, then learning that the patient was injured while being moved, or knowing a patient by sight, then learning that this patient has committed suicide—can result in feelings of "devastation" and "failure" among many staff members.[34] The word "devastating" also came up with respect to legal liability, both in terms of what being sued can do to one's career and in terms of "the folk wisdom" among physicians concerning the percentage of patients who do sue.[35] Given this snapshot of the psychological and spiritual dimensions of how medical harm is experienced by clinicians, it is not surprising to learn that, according to a director of pastoral care who also serves as a medical school instructor and chaplain, "theological concepts can be useful even if you don't use [theological] language" when counseling clinicians after critical incidents.[36]

Although there is virtually no literature on the role of professional hospital chaplains in providing emotional support to medical students, physicians, and other clinicians after medical mistakes, these and other conversations indicate that some chaplains are regularly involved in counseling clinicians after mistakes, and that chaplains in general view the provision of pastoral care to hospital staff as a "recognized part of [their] ministry."[37] A chaplain who had previously worked as a nurse for more than 30 years said she could imagine creating a "ritual of forgiveness" on her unit to help hospital staff come to terms with their own errors: "I could picture me doing it—I don't think it's far-fetched at all."[38] However, what is true for the M&M hair-shirt ritual is also true for any alternative rituals that are practiced or being developed elsewhere within hospital culture. The injured patient is not a member of these "congregations." As such, these rituals do not provide the patient with an opportunity to forgive if he chooses to do so, because they do not ensure that the patient has first received justice.

And what might the justice-making project encompass following medical harm? Recalling the recovered Jewish tradition of *tikkun olam*, with its underlying image of the repair of a shattered world and its attentiveness to the social context of justice, the concluding chapter of this book consists of some practical suggestions derived from the needs, concerns, and cautions identified in the previous chapters. This is not intended as an all-or-nothing list of ethical responses to medical harm, but aims to describe practices that can be incorporated into the cultures of community hospitals and university medical centers alike — and that, for the most part, do not cost the institution anything to implement. Even the proposal that hospitals provide fair compensation to injured patients is cost-effective, when weighed against the costs of litigation. In their frequently cited analysis of the financial impact of the Lexington Model of full disclosure, discussed in the previous chapter, Steve S. Kraman and Ginny Hamm observed that the policy had "resulted in unanticipated financial benefits" due to the decrease in legal and administrative costs incurred in defending malpractice suits, and concluded that "an honest and forthright risk management policy that puts the patient's interests first may be relatively inexpensive."[39]

The assignment of suggested practices into the traditional Western religious categories of "confession," "repentance," and "forgiveness" is necessarily subjective. In general, practices listed under "confession" involve truth telling, apology, and other communications between those held accountable for medical harm and those who have suffered as the result of medical harm. Practices listed under "repentance" include actions that those held accountable may take following the disclosure of medical harm to ensure that any medical, financial, or other needs of injured patients and families are addressed. Practices listed under "forgiveness" may be thought of as existing in *kairos* time, in that they are envisioned as taking place whenever appropriate, which may mean "often," "all the time," or "before the next patient is injured."

In the cheap-grace material that introduces *Discipleship*, Bonhoeffer excoriates institutions that seek to protect themselves at the expense of justice. To create patient-safety systems that acknowledge the suffering and protect the interests of injured patients and their families, allowing them to detach and to forgive, administrators, clinicians, educators, and others involved in patient-safety efforts within health care institutions must learn to be ever attentive to Bonhoeffer's "view from below," which is always in the first instance the perspective of the harmed patient and family. In so doing, they may avoid the cheap grace of presuming that it is enough for the institution to confess to and to forgive itself, for harms done to those in its care.

CHAPTER EIGHT

Ethical Action

There are ways to improve how individuals working within systems care for injured patients and their families and for clinicians whose mistakes harm patients. In the proposals that follow, I draw on the religious and cultural traditions that have helped to shape secular Western norms and expectations surrounding error and forgiveness, while looking critically at these traditions, their limits, and the ways they can be used against the interests of those who suffer. This is not an all-or-nothing list. There are many different kinds of medical mistakes, many different kinds of health care institutions, and many different ways that such institutions can respond, concretely and compassionately, to the needs of all parties affected by medical mistakes. Although these proposals reinforce the recommendations included in the preceding chapters, they are intended to provide further opportunities for productive discussion and action.

The practices traditionally described as confession, and encompassing truth telling and apology, include:

- Promptly acknowledging error and disclosing to the injured patient a cogent and complete narrative of what happened.

The issue that physicians call "disclosure" and patients and families call "being told what happened" is perhaps the most contentious and emotionally fraught aspect of the aftermath of medical harm. It might seem that suing and being sued would claim this dubious honor. However, personal narratives, plus a growing number of experiential accounts of disclosure practices within health care systems, confirm that telling or not telling patients the truth about what happened to their bodies — or, in the case of families, their loved ones' lives — is the hinge on which all else hangs: apology for harm, accountability for preventing further mistakes, compensation and how it will be secured, and the ability to gain some psychological distance from a traumatic episode in one's life, and to go forward, or to be bound forever to that trauma.

If everything else flows from telling injured patients and their families the truth, what, in Bonhoeffer's phrase, is meant by "telling" the truth? Keeping the focus on the "telling" may help physicians to get past one frequently voiced objection: the absolute "truth" may not be knowable. Theologians and postmodern philosophers alike will agree with this sentiment, arguing, respectively, that absolute truth is unknowable by human beings, or that there is no such thing as absolute truth, only multiple truth claims. However, medical error, like all human error, happens in the realm of the quotidian and the earth-bound. If the capital-T Truth about human existence remains a mystery, uncovering the facts about a given incident, interpreting those facts with reference to the standards and practices of the culture in which the incident took place, and describing these activities in a way that can be understood by persons inside and outside that culture, is something that human beings do, or attempt to do, all the time. Physicians make do with small-t truth every time they take a patient's history, propose a diagnosis, or recommend a course of treatment. Omniscience is not a human characteristic, but it is intellectually dishonest for physicians, or anyone else, to claim that because all cannot be known, nothing can be known, and therefore nothing can be told.

Moreover, physicians' own professional culture teaches them something about the "telling" part of "telling the truth" about their mistakes, through their participation in the Morbidity and Mortality Conference, a forum where confessions are regularly heard but, as Atul Gawande points out, cannot be used as evidence of liability.[1] Gawande also notes that M&M, as a professional ritual within the culture of medicine, has a normative and a descriptive function. It is not sufficient to tell your colleagues what you did wrong; you must also tell them what you ought to have done (Gawande 2002, 62).

Gawande contends that it is "almost impossible" for physicians to honor their truth-telling obligations to injured patients and blames "hospital lawyers" (Gawande 2002, 57) for this quandary. But is this really a fair claim? It is certainly true that hospital attorneys and risk managers have traditionally advised physicians to be parsimonious with the information they disclose to patients about errors. It is likely that these professional cultures are experiencing their own difficulties in absorbing research findings and other experiential data, strongly suggesting that a 180-degree shift in policy and practice, from nondisclosure to full disclosure, may be a better way to protect health care institutions and individual physicians from lawsuits. Yet if every hospital attorney and risk manager were suddenly to follow the lead of the lawyers and risk managers at the Lexington VAMC, Catholic Healthcare West, and COPIC, and start advising physicians that the *best* way to protect themselves from lawsuits was to promptly and fully disclose mistakes to patients in ways that patients can understand, would physicians follow their advice?

One physician, speaking from the anonymity of a focus group, acknowledges implicitly that the stereotype of the "hospital lawyer" as the sole barrier to disclosure may be a bit out of date: "everything you read and everything that you're told says that you are supposed to tell what errors you make as soon as you can . . . the question is, how many of us believe that?"[2] As long as physicians fear what injured patients and their families can do to their reputations, their finances, and their livelihoods, they are unlikely to "believe" any evidence suggesting that telling the truth is the best way to protect themselves from what they fear most.

If physicians are not yet ready to "believe" that honoring the obligation to disclose mistakes is a smart move in terms of self-protection, ethical arguments for disclosure that are based on appeals to professional obligations may fail to have the desired effect. Physicians have written about the central importance of recognizing that telling the truth after medical mistakes is part of a physician's role responsibility, because a mistake is part of the health information patients are entitled to receive from their physicians.[3] However, there is latitude to maneuver here for physicians who want to believe that they are upstanding members of their profession but do not really want to disclose mistakes or, at least, to disclose them so that patients understand that they are being told about a mistake and what the ramifications of that mistake are. One physician in the same focus-group study captured, perhaps unconsciously, the seductiveness of equivocation: "I think you have to be a spin doctor all the time and put the right spin on it . . . I don't think you have to soft pedal the issue, but I think you have to put it in the best light. I think you have to be forthright with patients to help them. And how you word it makes a big difference."[4] Alas, "spin doctor" does not happily coexist with "forthright." A physician who is preoccupied with spinning the truth is not having an honest conversation with his patient, even though he may believe that he is.

If appeals to research findings and to professional ethics should fail to persuade many physicians to disclose their mistakes, the appeal to narrative ethics remains. It is still uncommon for physicians and hospital administrators to hear injured patients or their families tell their stories outside of an adversarial context, or for published versions of their stories to be taught in medical school or discussed among clinicians. Virtually every one of these stories stresses the importance of maintaining honest communication between physician and patient and describes the painful consequences that result when a physician or an institution breaks off communication with an injured patient, or with a family after a patient's death. It is hard to read or listen to these stories and not be moved, not to question one's resistance to responding to the one who is in concrete distress. During grand rounds, a second-year resident heard a reading of Sandra Gilbert's story about the surgeon who told her, quite sincerely, that her husband's death was "unpleasant" for her, but "*shattering*" for him.[5] During the discussion period, the resident began with the familiar refrain of resistance: there's no way to know what the Truth is about what happened to this patient, so how can we expect the surgeon to tell it? But then the resident added, "I can't believe he *said* that," his disgusted tone indicating not that he doubted Gilbert's account of the surgeon's cold comfort, but rather that he was appalled by it. In his resistance, he was touched, as a professional and as a human being, by the story itself. Narratives of medical harm, when incorporated into medical school curricula and into grand rounds and other professional education opportunities for residents and senior physicians, have the power to serve as an antidote to the lessons of the hidden curriculum regarding disclosure and as a corrective to stereotypes concerning "angry" patients and families. Such narratives, when incorporated into forums in which patients and families affected by medical mistakes may interact with health care professionals, may similarly have the power to counteract the demonization of physicians who make mistakes.

- Apologizing and expressing remorse to injured patients — and allowing oneself to feel remorse after harming a patient.

Offering an apology should be part of the disclosure of a harmful medical mistake. An apology signifies to patients and families that the responsible party acknowledges and regrets the injury and other suffering that has resulted from such a mistake. In addition to being simple good manners, an apology may be deeply important to a patient or family, who may otherwise feel "abandoned and aggrieved" by their ostensible caregivers: as Carol Levine writes about the aftermath of the error that cost her husband his right hand, "he had suffered a terrible loss and no one seemed to care."[6]

As discussed in chapter 5, physicians may still be reluctant to offer an apology and admit fault if they believe that to say "I'm sorry" is to open themselves up to litigation; health care institutions may, for the same reason, still instruct physicians not to apologize or otherwise acknowledge personal responsibility. Yet the narratives of injured patients and their families, and the positive experiences of health care institutions that have integrated apology into the disclosure of medical mistakes, make it increasingly difficult to defend the notion that offering a sincere apology for a known mistake is somehow a bad idea.

Offering a sincere apology may also help the physician who is grappling with her own feelings about having harmed a patient while trying to help that patient. In his account of a mistaken diagnosis that led to the termination of a viable and wanted pregnancy, physician David Hilfiker writes, "Although mistakes are not usually sins, they engender similar feelings of guilt. How can I not feel guilty about the death of Barb's baby . . . ? Whether I 'ought' to feel guilty is a moot point; most of us do feel guilty under such circumstances."[7] Saying "I'm sorry" — and meaning it, and accepting the full consequences of these words — is a time-honored way to expiate paralyzing feelings of guilt or shame that a psychologically healthy person feels after having unintentionally harmed another person. Legal reforms that would protect the physician who says "I'm sorry" may be one way to encourage sincere apologies. But these are hard words to say, and physicians may need training, guidance, and institutional support in learning how to speak them.

- Being personally accountable even in cases of systems error, bearing in mind that some patients may comprehend error in all cases as an individual rather than a collective or systemic failure.

An unfortunate, at times convenient or legalistic, but wholly foreseeable reduction of the debate over individual versus systems accountability for medical error runs something like this: if experts now agree it's the "system's" fault, I'm off the hook, right? Such reasoning is bound to be unsatisfying, even suspect, to patients and families affected by medical mistakes if offered as an "explanation" for such mistakes. Some patients and families may also object in principle to the concept of "systems error," arguing that only individuals have moral agency, and therefore, only individuals can make mistakes and be responsible for the consequences of these mistakes. This position is not quite the same as holding individual "bad apples" responsible for mistakes. Rather, it is a resistance to any idea of collective responsibility that does not adequately hold individuals responsible for actions that could have been set in motion only by these individuals.[8]

Relying on "the system" as an explanation for medical error is probably going to be unsatisfying to many physicians as well, whether because they know that physicians, owing to their role responsibilities and decision-making authority, are bound to be involved in most medical mistakes in some way, or because they are individuals caring for other individuals, and invoking "the system" when their well-intentioned actions inadvertently harm patients simply feels wrong.

"The system" may provide the context for a medical mistake, but does not, in and of itself, provide an adequate explanation for a mistake. Personal accountability to individuals affected by medical mistakes can and should coexist with the system's ability to investigate, identify, and correct systems errors and to address the concrete needs of affected parties.

- Providing opportunities for clinicians to explore and resolve their emotional responses to harmful mistakes in an environment that is neither punitive nor demeaning.

It is difficult to imagine anyone in contemporary medicine who would argue in favor of the traditional "blame-and-shame" approach to the aftermath of medical error, which holds that mistakes are made by "bad apples" who can be isolated and punished. Yet rooting out the remnants of blaming and shaming attitudes within professional and institutional cultures continues to be a challenge for physicians and others involved in patient-safety efforts. In this, medicine is no different from society in general. It's easier, and perhaps more satisfying psychologically, to pin blame on an individual rather than to do the hard work of facing and addressing systems problems.

Consider Shirley Jackson's classic story, "The Lottery," which describes an annual ritual in an American small town. Each summer, the members of the community gather on the village green. The name of one member of the community is drawn from an ancient wooden box, and that person is immediately stoned to death by her family and friends. When we read this story, usually as high school students, the question that comes to mind is, why doesn't anyone ever move away? What keeps them in such a horrifying place, where they risk death at the hands of their neighbors each year? The answer, of course, is the utility of scapegoating. The lottery functions as a powerful expiation and identity ritual for the entire community. If your name does not come up, you are licensed to project your individual and collective demons onto your unfortunate neighbor, to get rid of them by destroying her, and to go home satisfied that you have once again driven out evil from your midst. Then, it's business as usual until next summer. Do this enough times, and you don't even have to think about what you are doing, because it is simply "what's done."

A less extreme example of institutionalized blaming and shaming can be found in Kathleen Norris's *Dakota*, her autobiographical account of contemporary life in a Great Plains community so small that the title of one chapter is "Can you tell the truth in a small town?"⁹ As Norris writes, "We don't tend to see the truth as something that could set us free because it means embracing pain, acknowledging our differences and conflicts, taking our real situation into account" (Norris 1993, 82). In her town, and in other communities in the region, the turnover of "teachers, doctors, and clergy" never ceased, due to the use of blaming and shaming by longtime community members as a substitute for facing problems or addressing the need to improve the performance of their institutions and not unlike the residents of the fictional village in "The Lottery," as a means of affirming the "unity" of those who remained (Norris 1993, 59). She quotes one pastor who says of his own nearby town, "it seems like every year somebody gets crucified" (Norris 1993, 59).

Health care institutions are not unlike small towns in this respect. Blaming and shaming is ultimately toxic to a culture — Norris describes a community caught in a blame-and-shame cycle as a place that "seems to have fallen under an evil spell" (Norris 1993, 59) — but in the short term it is also psychologically cathartic, even addictive, and may appear to be effective. Most human beings like tidy endings to their stories, and getting rid of a "bad apple" — or "crucifying" a "bad" doctor — is seductive as a fantasy of resolution. Efforts to replace blaming and shaming with "systems approaches" to resolving errors are unlikely to be effective if they fail to take these powerful and not always articulated functions of blaming and shaming into account.

Systems approaches to improving the handling of medical mistakes should also attempt to help clinicians avoid internalized blaming and shaming in the aftermath of mistakes. Researchers have found that mere slogans about "blame-free" approaches to patient safety had no effect on the "anguish and sense of culpability for errors" among the physicians they studied.[10] These researchers recommend that health care institutions "assess and support the emotional needs of practitioners as an explicit component of every error analysis" and suggest that "[b]etter institutional support for caregivers involved in errors" will result in better care for injured patients, because physicians will be less likely to be overwhelmed by their own emotions in the aftermath of their mistakes and better able to perceive and respond to the needs of their patients.[11]

Within institutions, who should provide such care to physicians and other clinicians after they make mistakes? Professional chaplains may function as counselors for some physicians following errors or other traumatic incidents, whereas other physicians rely on their peers. These "confessions," however, may be less than complete, and the degree of emotional support offered may vary greatly. As physician Albert Wu writes, after a physician makes a mistake, "reassurance from colleagues is often grudging or qualified," and "confession is discouraged, passively by lack of appropriate forums for discussion, and sometimes actively by risk managers and hospital lawyers."[12] Wu proposes a more engaged form of peer support in which colleagues would encourage one another to fully describe and acknowledge their mistakes and follow up by "ask[ing] how the colleague is coping" (Wu 2000, 727). Other professionals familiar with the culture of health care institutions propose the creation of a "confessor" function within hospitals, with this role to be played by a "colleague knowledgeable about error" who stood outside of the supervision or evaluation of individual clinicians.[13] None of these proposals is perfect, and no single proposal is likely to work for every type of health care institution.[14] However, each of these proposals offers a way to subvert the blame-and-shame cycle within institutions and individuals by tapping into deeply rooted normative practices of listening and being listened to, practices that may fulfill and supplant the cathartic and ritual functions of blaming- and-shaming activities.

- Nurturing as a communal principle within health care institutions that withholding the truth violates patient autonomy and has a corrosive effect on caregivers.

Over the past 20 years, the codes of the American Medical Association and the American College of Physicians have adopted language that identifies truth telling after medical error as a professional obligation for all physicians.[15,16] In 2001, the Joint Commission on the Accreditation of Healthcare Organizations, the accrediting body for more than 5,000 hospitals in the United States, added disclosure of "unanticipated outcomes," including errors, to its patient-safety standards.[17] Drawing individual physicians' attention to their professional truth-telling obligations is important. Drawing hospital leaders' attention to their organizational truth-telling obligations is important. But educational efforts around these themes, which are ongoing in the peer-to-peer literature and throughout the patient-safety movement, must be supported by actual practices within health care institutions. The need for professional and corporate values to be enacted daily in practice is especially acute in teaching hospitals, where the influence of the hidden curriculum may quickly cause medical students and residents to "unlearn" what they were taught about the centrality of truth telling within the physician-patient relationship, particularly if the disclosure of medical error was never identified and taught as a truth-telling practice in the first place.

Recalling Bonhoeffer's description of truth telling as an ethical practice in which "speaking" is the action, one might conclude, particularly if one has done, or failed to do, something that one is not anxious to disclose, that "not speaking" is not an action and cannot therefore be described in terms of its ethics. In her magisterial study of "the ethics of concealment and revelation," Sissela Bok addresses the ethics of not speaking the truth.[18] While allowing that secrecy is indeed distinct from lying, which she describes as *"prima facie* wrong," (Bok 1982, xv), Bok argues that practices associated with secrecy, including not speaking the truth, can indeed be assessed in terms of their ethics. Bok sees notable peril in "long-term group practices of secrecy": "[These practices] are especially likely to breed corruption and to spread. Every aspect of the shared predicament influences the secret practice cumulatively over time: in particular, the impediments to reasoning and to choice, and the limitations on sympathy and on regard for human beings. The tendency to view the world in terms of insiders and outsiders can then build up a momentum that it would lack if it were short-lived and immediately accountable" (Bok 1982, 110). When a professional or an institutional culture within health care values the practice of secrecy over the practice of candor in the aftermath of mistakes that harm those in its care, this practice effectively cancels out the notion of physician-patient communication. As Bok notes, the freedom to keep the secret constrains the freedom of those who are denied the information being kept secret (Bok 1982, 26). And by perpetuating the notion of injured patients and their families as a category of persons to whom accurate and complete information about their own health and well-being is not owed, physicians and hospital administrators, in effect, blame and shame those patients and families who have the audacity to demand to know what really happened. This may, in turn, contribute to a certain hardening of caregivers' attitudes toward injured patients and their legitimate requests.

It is difficult to imagine that physicians, even in their deepest moments of fear concerning the potential repercussions of disclosing their mistakes, view scapegoating injured patients and their families for the sin of wanting to know what happened as an ethically appropriate response to medical harm. Yet without sustained attention, by professional organizations, by medical educators, and, most important, within individual health care institutions and their subcultures, to the ways in which actual truth-telling practices fall short of or sabotage professional and corporate obligations, the blame-and-shame culture, a culture which refuses to tell itself the truth, will continue to harm patients and families as well as clinicians and institutions.[19]

• Avoiding the scapegoating of subordinates.

Patient-safety advocate Roxanne Goeltz tells a story about the hospital CEO who is asked how he finds out when a medical error has taken place at his institution. "When we fire a nurse," he replies.[20] Although this story may or may not be apocryphal, like many such stories it contains a kernel of truth about the culture in which it is set. Nurses may be treated more harshly than physicians when both bear some responsibility for the same mistake, and the immense difference in status between physicians and all other clinicians may lead to the scapegoating of less powerful members of the hierarchy. It is for these reasons that Catholic Healthcare West's "Philosophy of Mistake Management" recognizes the "perceived or actual difference between the status of physicians and nurses," and states that "both will be treated equitably" in the aftermath of mistakes.[21]

Analogous possibilities for scapegoating actual or perceived subordinates in the aftermath of medical harm exist between more senior physicians and more junior physicians or residents ("it's always the resident who gets flayed for the screwups"),[22] between residents and students; and between different medical specialties. Hospitals are hierarchies, and in a hierarchy it is so easy and so tempting to take advantage of the inherent imbalances of power by "firing a nurse," literally or figuratively, rather than making certain that all parties who bear some responsibility for a mistake are identified and all circumstances that contributed to the error are brought to light. Because of this constant temptation, health care institutions should build and enforce specific protections against scapegoating into their policies, practices, and training relevant to the aftermath of medical error.

- Avoiding the abuse of the unequal distribution of power between a physician and an injured patient, which may be further skewed by gender, race, income, age, culture, disability, or a combination of these or other factors. Relevant abuses of authority would include making a patient complicit in a known or suspected error by labeling her "noncompliant"; conflating harm with "complications" or other terms that may be used to conceal mistakes; or taking advantage of a patient's religious beliefs — "It was God's will" — to conceal or minimize error.

Physicians may think of themselves as less powerful than injured patients and their families if they have been taught to view such patients and families as angry adversaries and potential litigants. But in the physician-patient relationship, the physician is always the more powerful actor, whether or not she is comfortable with that role. The injured patient, moreover, has been rendered more, not less, vulnerable as the result of his injury. Already vulnerable as the result of illness or other impairment, he has been harmed by those whom he entrusted to help him. Keeping these uncomfortable truths in mind may help physicians to respond to injured patients and their families with humility and compassion rather than fear and suspicion. Physicians should also be mindful of the terms they may use, at times almost reflexively, to characterize patients, families, or clinical situations, as certain words and phrases, although arguably appropriate in some circumstances, can be inappropriate, unjust, and even dangerous when error is known or suspected.

In *The Spirit Catches You and You Fall Down: A Hmong Child, Her American Doctors, and the Collision between Two Cultures,* journalist Anne Fadiman tells the story of Lia Lee, a little girl with severe epilepsy, and the clash between the way her family's animist culture understood her condition and the way it was understood by the physicians at Merced Community Medical Center (MCMC) in California's Central Valley, where the Lees had been resettled after the Vietnam War and a decade in a refugee camp in Thailand.[23] Compliance with Lia's complicated and ever-changing medication regimen was a constant source of tension in the relationship between Lia's family, to whom the concept of preventive medicine was culturally foreign, and her primary doctors, a married couple named Neil Ernst and Peggy Philp, who feared that "the big one" — an uncontrollable seizure —

would inevitably result (Fadiman 1997, 143). After "the big one," which did indeed take place and caused irreversible brain damage to Lia, Fadiman interviewed a neurologist at another hospital where Lia had been treated. This physician told Fadiman that septic shock, not undermedication, caused Lia's final seizure, and that her most recent medication, which had immunosuppressant properties, might even have "set her up" for an infection (Fadiman 1997, 255). He recommended that she "Go back to Merced . . . and tell all those people at MCMC that the family didn't do this to the kid. We did" (Fadiman 1997, 255). When Fadiman tells them of this neurologist's opinion, Neil Ernst and Peggy Philp are amazed that they overlooked the possibility of septic shock as the trigger for the catastrophic seizure. One of their colleagues was not as surprised: "If Neil made a mistake, it's because every physician makes mistakes. If it had been a brand-new [patient] . . . I guarantee you Neil would have done a septic workup and he would have caught it. But this was Lia. *No one* at MCMC would have noticed anything but her seizures. Lia *was* her seizures" (Fadiman 1997, 256).

And because "Lia *was* her seizures," parental noncompliance with her antiseizure medication regimen had to be the reason for all her health problems, including "the big one" that her physicians were dreading. Commitment to "noncompliance" as an all-purpose explanation meant that they simply could not see other possibilities, including their own possible error in medication choice. It is all too easy to see how the word "noncompliance" — a word that clinicians, not patients, are allowed to use, and which, as Arthur Kleinman notes, implies a moral defect on the part of the patient — could be used in other cases, consciously or unconsciously, to deflect responsibility for an error from a "good" doctor to a "bad" patient.[24]

"Complications" is another term that can be misused, consciously or unconsciously, to conceal error, whether from the patient or from the physician himself. For example, in a journal article entitled "I Wish Things Were Different," physicians Timothy E. Quill, Robert M. Arnold, and Frederick Platt offer their peers a number of "sample responses" to help them communicate with patients in clinical situations of "loss, futility, or unrealistic hopes."[25] The authors characterize "responding to medical complications *or errors*" as a single "representative clinical scenario," although elsewhere in the article they do distinguish between complications and errors.[26] Of course, in the clinical setting and in other professions, an error *is* a complication. But using the word "complication" as a substitute for "error" when communicating with a patient or family member — or indeed, anyone else — is disingenuous. Telling an injured patient or family member that "there's been a complication" is not the same as disclosing an error; rather than fulfilling a physician's obligation to tell the truth, this phrase disguises the truth in a way that a layperson may be unlikely to question. And, as with the word "noncompliance," the word "complication" can shift scrutiny and responsibility away from the physician. No one "makes" a complication.

During the past decade, "cultural competency" has been integrated into medical education. Medical students and residents have been taught that part of being a good doctor is knowing something of the culture of the communities they serve and respecting, as much as possible, the cultural beliefs, values, and practices of individual patients. Cultural competency is a worthy goal, but appealing to a patient's known or presumed religious beliefs or cultural norms for the purpose of concealing error is not. The following story, told by a plaintiff's attorney and included in Sandra Gilbert's *Wrongful Death*, illustrates how one physician tried to do just that:

> A guy from down the Peninsula came to me. Wealthy man, good Catholic. A big contributor to a Catholic hospital down there. A *patron*, a benefactor. And his wife went in there for routine surgery . . . Came out of the OR in a coma. Lived for a month or two in a nursing home, then passed away . . . Happens all the time . . . But the doctor could have leveled, could have made it better. This man and the doctor, they belong to the same club in San Francisco. The guy takes the doctor out to lunch at the club once, twice. Each time, he looks at the doctor and says, "What happened, Doc? What happened to my Mary?" "I don't know," says the doctor. "'It was God's will, Frank. These things are mysterious. Who knows what happened. It was God's will." . . . God's will! Well, the man came to *me*, had to find out what happened to his wife. And we deposed the people who were in the OR, found out what everyone knew all along. The perfusion machine — that's a machine that keeps the patient breathing during the surgery — ran out of oxygen. Someone just forgot to fill it. And you only have two minutes in a situation like that, then she's brain dead. Comes out of there comatose . . . Happens all the time. But this guy was a good Catholic, a patron of the hospital. If the doctor had leveled with him, he wouldn't have sued.[27]

This physician hoped that by invoking the phrase "God's will," he could shame a devout Catholic into not asking any more questions. He also believed that by not telling the truth about what happened, not "leveling," he could prevent a lawsuit. He was wrong on both counts. In certain circumstances — in Lia Lee's case, for example — it may be appropriate and even desirable for a physician to demonstrate some understanding of a patient's culture or beliefs, to enhance physician-patient communications, and to redistribute the imbalance of power between them. But it is never appropriate for a physician to use a patient's beliefs against a patient's own interests, including coercive appeals to a patient's presumed beliefs to hide mistakes or discourage questions.

The practice traditionally described as repentance includes:
- Not forcing the patient to interact with the person responsible for her injury if the patient does not wish to do so.

Looking at the aftermath of medical harm from the perspective of the injured patient means honoring that patient's feelings concerning the parties responsible for her injury, and her beliefs concerning the act of truth telling. Some patients simply may not want to be in the same room with the physician whose mistake harmed them, particularly if there was not a strong or satisfactory level of communication between this physician and the patient prior to the incident. Some patients may value an explanation and apology from the hospital's chief executive or medical director, rather than from the clinicians directly responsible for their injuries, if they are especially concerned about institutional accountability. In neither of these cases would it be appropriate to restore physician-patient communications in principle by forcing the injured patient into a conversation he does not want to have, or into a role that is distressing or unsatisfactory to him. Rather, honoring the patient's perspective requires responsible parties to listen to the patient, rather than merely writing him into the script.

In the medical ethics literature, there are several well-known exceptions to the principle that respecting patient autonomy with regard to truth telling means that physicians should provide information directly to their patients, rather than through surrogates. When the patient is a child, or mentally handicapped, or unconscious, or does not speak the same language as the physician, or has a psychiatric disorder, or comes from a culture whose norms concerning truth telling may preclude breaking bad news directly to certain categories of persons, health information may be disclosed to a family member or other surrogate. After such a patient has been injured through error, the obligation to disclose remains in effect despite the presence of a barrier to direct disclosure. As Ginny Hamm and Steve Kraman of the Lexington VAMC write, exceptions to direct disclosure "should be based on the impact to the patient and family and not to relieve the obligation" of responsible parties, and decisions to disclose errors by means of surrogates should not rest with individual clinicians, but should involve the hospital's ethics committee as well.[28]

It is striking that the Lexington Model of disclosure, as practiced by the

Lexington VAMC itself, does not require individual physicians to disclose their own errors; this institution argues that "the ethical obligation is institutional," in part because of the systems dimension of most errors, in part because most physicians employed by the VAMC are residents.[29] As a result physicians who are in general agreement with the Lexington Model have criticized this aspect of it on several grounds.[30] Exempting residents from the duty to disclose their own mistakes alienates them from their professional obligations. Institutionally, a teachable moment is lost when a teaching institution does not give its residents the opportunity to learn how to disclose their own mistakes, a lesson that they will surely need to draw on throughout their careers.[31] And transferring responsibility for disclosure to another party, without considering the wishes of the injured patient or the patient's family, once again neglects the patient's perspective. At the Lexington VAMC, physicians whose mistakes resulted in harm are "always welcome to be part of the disclosure" and subsequent meetings with injured patients.[32] It is not that difficult to imagine an improvement to this admirable model by ensuring that patients and families are similarly "always welcome" to request that all responsible parties take part in the disclosure pro cess.

- Appreciating the difference between appropriate feelings of guilt ("I made a mistake") and destructive feelings of shame ("I am a mistake").

According to a hospital chaplain who teaches medical ethics and has counseled medical students and physicians in the aftermath of errors, "I made a mistake" is an "appropriate" way to acknowledge one's personal responsibility for an error; "I am a mistake" is not.[33] After making a mistake that has harmed a patient — or even after a near miss or "harmless hit" — a clinician may feel that he should never touch another patient. A nurse recalls a shift early in her training when she missed a ward while delivering medications. After she discovered her mistake, she felt "demoralized, worthless, stupid."[34] In her own eyes, *she* became the mistake, and her supervisor "had to work with me to get me to do meds again."[35] As this clinician learned, shame can be paralyzing, even when, as in this case, a mistake does not harm a single patient. And making a mistake that does harm a patient is not an event that can be lightly brushed off. Nor should it be — feeling and working through *normal* guilt, as opposed to crippling shame, is what distinguishes a psychologically healthy individual from a psychopath. Feeling guilty about mistakes, responding to these feelings constructively by identifying and correcting problems, and being ever aware of one's own fallibility may also protect clinicians from rationalizing their own errors. Writing about his own spe-cialty, Atul Gawande notes: "There are surgeons who will see faults everywhere except in themselves. They have no questions and no fears about their abilities. As a result, they learn nothing from their mistakes and know nothing of their limitations. As one surgeon told me, it is a rare but alarming thing to meet a surgeon without fear. 'If you're not a little afraid when you operate,' he said, 'you're bound to do a patient a grave disservice'" (Gawande 2002, 61).

•   Offering injured patients and their families access to mental health ser-vices should they desire them.

The stories that patients, family members, and physicians write about the aftermath of medical errors attest to the profound emotional toll of these errors. With respect to the specific needs of patients and families, hospital administra-tors should examine their disclosure policies and practices to ensure that patients and families receive adequate emotional support throughout the disclosure pro-cess and should talk with patients and families affected by medical mistakes at their institutions to obtain their perspectives on what was helpful, what could have been improved, what was lacking, and what was harmful in the institution's handling of the mistake.

When writing for their peers, physicians will often compare the act of disclos-ing medical error to "breaking bad news," a professional obligation that no physician enjoys but that all are expected to learn and perform throughout their careers.[36] In some hospitals, chaplains are in the room when patients are receiv-ing bad news, particularly when no other family members are present.[37] Al-though the patient's physician is responsible for the actual communication — which may involve confirming a diagnosis, telling the patient that a treatment has not been successful, or that curative options have been exhausted — the chaplain is responsible for providing emotional support to the patient and family, in some cases simply by being present and available.

If disclosing medical error is similar to breaking bad news from the perspec-tive of the physician's professional duties, and if being present when bad news is delivered is often part of the hospital chaplain's professional duties, it is reason-able for hospitals to consider a role for professional chaplains — health care pro-fessionals with postgraduate theological and clinical training who function as members of the clinical care team — in the process by which confirmed errors are disclosed to patients and families. To do so is *not* to make chaplains into surro-gates for physicians concerning the disclosure of medical mistakes, but rather to draw on the chaplain's particular skills and experience in providing support to patients and families who are receiving distressing information.

Among health care professionals, hospital chaplains often go unrecognized as potential resources for health care institutions attempting to improve the care of persons affected by medical harm, while the topic of medical error has been absent from chaplains' own professional literature. Patient-safety organizations, chaplaincy-certifying organizations, and individual hospitals would do well, as a first step, to educate chaplains about medical error, integrate chaplains into institutional patient-safety efforts, and propose ways for chaplains to contribute insights from their profession to the development of disclosure processes that are attentive to the emotional toll of disclosure on patients and families — and on clinicians who are disclosing their own mistakes.

Beyond the immediate circumstances of the disclosure, it is possible that a patient or a patient's family may require more extensive therapeutic counseling after the disclosure of a mistake that leads to death or serious injury because of the sheer magnitude of the trauma. Given that hospitals employ many types of mental health professionals, it is tempting to suggest that hospitals ought to offer these professional services directly to patients and families. However, to avoid potential conflicts of interest with respect to a counselor's responsibilities to injured patients and their families, the counselor's collegial relationships with clinicians involved in medical mistakes, and even the counselor's perceptions of what the institution may desire as a therapeutic outcome — namely, that the patient or family will not file a lawsuit — it is more appropriate for the hospital to provide reimbursement for the cost of counseling by a professional who is not employed by or otherwise affiliated with the institution where the mistake took place.

Given that the status of counseling records under "health privacy" policies or statutes is not always clear, health care institutions could, in theory, subpoena an injured patient's counseling records if the patient decides to pursue a lawsuit and seek pain and suffering damages on the grounds of emotional distress.[38] As such, patients and families should be informed, ideally by their own legal counsel, as to how to protect the privacy of their counseling records, and health care institutions should forego the opportunity to subpoena such records even if they are legally permitted to do so.

Advocates and critics of mediation as an alternative to litigation often point out that there is a strong therapeutic dimension to this process. To some mediators, this is part of its appeal: "while mediation is not an intentionally therapeutic process, its practice and results are often similar to therapeutic interventions."[39]

To other mediators, advocating mediation because it is in some respects like therapy means that mediators must be aware of what goes on between therapist and client in an actual therapeutic setting. Mediators are supposed to be honest brokers, but, as mediator and law professor Trina Grillo argues, therapists are trained to be aware and make use of transference and countertransference, the ways in which the past experiences of the client and therapist, respectively, are inevitably reflected in the present-day therapeutic encounter.[40] Although "countertransference and transference also occur in mediation," they may go unrecognized or unacknowledged, to the potential detriment of the client (Grillo 1991, 22).[41] Although mediation may indeed be an effective tool for restoring communications and productively addressing the concrete needs of patients, families, clinicians, and institutions in the aftermath of medical harm, it should not be confused with therapy or relied on to deliver therapeutic benefits.

- Covering the cost of treating injuries resulting from error, and meeting other concrete needs resulting from loss of income due to injury or death resulting from error.

Carol Levine characterizes the "professional discussion of medical error" as "oddly disembodied": "Medical error is more than an engineering problem, amenable to technological and 'systems' solutions. Policies put in place to reduce medical error also must address the financial and emotional needs of those who suffer great and often permanent harm" (Levine 2002, 237). The fair compensation programs of the Lexington VAMC, Catholic Healthcare West, and COPIC represent three different alternatives to the tort system that are proving to be cost effective, ethically responsible, and far less emotionally brutalizing than waging or defending a lawsuit. These alternatives to litigation are premised on disclosure: Rather than waiting to be sued, physicians and institutions must initiate the process of fair compensation by telling patients the truth about the injuries they have sustained.

- Working to create conditions that may allow injured patients and their families, at some point in *their* futures, to detach from the incident as a continuing source of pain, anger, and injustice, while recognizing that directly asking an injured patient for "forgiveness" may be oppressive or culturally inappropriate with respect to that patient.

In Jewish and Christian traditions concerning error and forgiveness, and in the many secular rituals — from the Mortality and Morbidity Conference, to how parents teach small children what they should do after they have made a mistake that hurts someone else — that have been influenced by this tradition, the rituals of confession, repentance, and forgiveness are understood as transactions between persons and as transactions that depend on words and actions. These verbal transactions are evident in the case of a three-year-old named Madeleine, whose five-year-old brother accidentally bonked her on the head while they were playing. After being comforted by her mother, Madeleine calmly told her brother, "You can apologize to me now, Tyler." And he did, and they went back to playing together.

If it is important for the person — even a three-year-old person — who has been harmed to hear the words "I'm sorry," might it also be important for the person whose actions caused the harm to hear the words "I forgive you?" Perhaps. But it is essential to keep in mind that an apology can take place as soon as it is evident that one person has been harmed by another person's mistake: the fact of the mistake is sufficient catalyst for the words, "I'm sorry." But it does not follow that the words "I'm sorry" are sufficient catalyst for the words, "I forgive you." This is not solely a verbal transaction, or solely a matter of reflexive etiquette along the lines of saying, "you're welcome" upon hearing the words "thank you." As feminist ethicists Pamela Cooper-White and Marie Fortune have argued, an ethic of "instant forgiveness" after harm is both seductive and inappropriate.[42] It is seductive, because it *seems* to be the "right," the "good," (and, often in the United States, the stereotypically "Christian") response to harm, even in the absence of an apology or any evidence of remorse. Persons of religious faith who have been affected by medical mistakes frequently struggle with internalized norms concerning what they perceive as their obligation to forgive the physician whose error harmed them, or to forgive the hospital administrators who refused to tell their family what happened. They may "forgive" so they can continue to live in the same community, go to the same doctor, use the same hospital. They may "forgive" because, in the absence of an explanation and an apology, it is the only way they can attempt to resolve the trauma of having been harmed. But this is what psychologists call pseudoforgiveness, because the trauma has not been resolved, either materially or psychologically, and thus merely saying "I forgive you" brings neither relief nor release.

The physician who does say "I'm sorry," who does explain what happened, and who is accountable for preventing similar harm to other patients, should therefore neither ask for forgiveness, nor expect to hear the words "I forgive you" from an injured patient or a family affected by this physician's mistake. Asking for forgiveness may be oppressive to a patient or family still grappling with the fact of the harm, the impact of the harm, and their response to the harm. Asking them, during a time of crisis and even bereavement, to offer a formulaic and possibly culturally unfamiliar response to make the physician feel better—or, perhaps, provide some reassurance that there will be no lawsuit—is simply too much to ask. And expecting injured patients or their families to offer forgiveness in the *absence* of disclosure, apology, or accountability is unforgivable.

The practices designed to create the appropriate conditions for forgiveness include:

- Inviting injured patients to be part of the hospital's quality improvement (QI) process, to allow them, if they wish, to take an active role in working with clinicians and administrators to create and sustain a culture of safety by sharing their experiences of medical harm and their perspectives on hospital culture and health care delivery. This is not to suggest that injured patients are responsible for participating in QI to prevent other patients from being harmed, or to solve systemic problems.

In its *National Agenda for Action: Patients and Families in Patient Safety*, the Patient and Family Advisory Council (PFAC) of the National Patient Safety Foundation states: "As the patient-safety movement gains momentum, it is clear that patients and families must be adequately integrated into the systems we are striving to change."[43] PFAC proposes many substantive roles for patients and families who have been affected by medical error to play within hospitals' quality improvement processes, and in undergraduate and continuing medical education. Given that institutional accountability for preventing future harms may be highly valued by some injured patients and their families, offering these patients and families the opportunity to take part in the improvement of health care delivery systems may be personally meaningful to these individuals, and may signal to others within the institution that the patients' and families' perspectives are a legitimate part of QI. However, patients and families concerned with institutional accountability are in no way obligated to take part in QI activities. Nor can any merely token involvement of patients and families in QI activities substitute for active and sustained collaboration among patients, families, clinicians, educators, and administrators.

- Offering a ritual or other forum for physicians and other caregivers to explore their emotions in the aftermath of medical error, as well as their obligations to affected patients and families.

Rituals may help members of a community to come to terms emotionally with traumatic events. Not all rituals can do this: whereas M&M is an authentic cultural ritual within medicine, it is not a ritual whose primary goal is to help participants address the emotional or the self-transcendent aspects of mistakes, though some participants may find it satisfying in this respect. Although clinicians and medical educators may develop alternative rituals for addressing these aspects of mistakes, and should be supported in their efforts to do so, it is also possible to envision adapting existing rituals within the culture of medicine to further assist physicians in addressing their own emotional needs and providing support to patients and families.

For example, some hospitals have rituals to honor the memories of patients who have died. Unlike most other cultural rituals within hospitals, these services are open to patients' families. At one university medical center, the monthly Service of Remembrance is designed in the first instance for families, who may request that clinicians who cared for their loved ones be invited to the service, and can also arrange to meet privately with clinicians after the service.[44] This institution has found that this ritual is especially meaningful to those clinicians who cared for a patient but were not on duty when that patient died. It is not too hard to imagine a similar ritual in which family members, clinicians, and even administrators come together to acknowledge and mourn a death resulting from a mistake. Even learning about an existing ritual such as this Service of Remembrance may create an opportunity for a group of caregivers to explore and discuss precisely that moment that may be most difficult for an individual clinician, grappling with the emotional fallout of a mistake, to imagine: a nonadversarial meeting with a family in the aftermath of medical harm. Other rituals within medicine, such as the "white coat" ceremony in which graduating medical students are invested with the emblem of their profession, could similarly be adapted to incorporate some reference to the fallibility as well as the power of the physician, as a reminder to young physicians that they should not and need not expect always to be responsible for healing themselves.

- Using ethics education opportunities within health care institutions to help clinicians, other health care professionals, and students to develop their capacity to understand medical harm from the patient's perspective; learn how to frame forgiveness after harm as detachment predicated on justice while recognizing non-Western paradigms of reconciliation or resolution after harm, and identifying and challenging any aspects of institutional culture that deny the fallibility, and therefore the humanity, of health care providers, or that work against the interests of injured patients and their families.

David Hilfiker begins his essay, "From the Victim's Point of View," by asking, "[w]hat does the ethicist ultimately want from health professionals and students? What is the goal of teaching and lecturing in ethics, of discussing and cajoling?"[45] He proposes that one goal of ethics education, one thing that the ethicist ought to want, is "to develop in those who care for others an empathy with the outsider, with the excluded, with the victim" (Hilfiker 2001, 255). This seems so obvious. Even Hilfiker acknowledges it really isn't asking too much of professional caregivers to expect them to feel empathy for those in their care. But when applied to the problem of medical harm, the fears and myths associated with injured patients and their "angry" families are such that it may be difficult for caregivers to recognize the injured patient—or the family of a patient who has died or been disabled following an error—as the ultimate "outsider."

The perspective that David Hilfiker—and Dietrich Bonhoeffer—propose as essential to the doing and teaching of ethics does not require every health care professional to take on the role of patient advocate in the aftermath of medical harm, but it does require every health care professional, in his or her own capacity, to work on behalf of the injured patient's interests. In addition to helping health care professionals think through what Hilfiker's challenge means with respect to how their own professions respond to the needs of injured patients and their families, ethics education around patient safety may help these professionals to confront and transcend the frequent, at times reflexive, response to error in the context of clinical medicine: "everyone makes mistakes." Yes, everyone does—to err is human—but this response is about the person who made the mistake, not about the persons who may have been harmed by the mistake, and it utterly fails to address the aftermath of harmful mistakes. If we agree that everyone makes mistakes, we are required, as rational and moral beings, to think about what happens next. If we acknowledge that our societal and professional norms value truth telling and fairness over secrecy and neglect, we are required to use these norms as guides to our actual behavior and practices in the aftermath of harm. If we value forgiveness as among the desirable responses to human error, we are required not to devalue it as cheap grace, but to recognize it as the final step in the process of helping those who suffer to detach from the trauma of having been harmed.

Reader's Guide

Paul B. Batalden, M.D., and Jeffrey L. Rice, M.D.

These questions were developed to provoke inquiry into the themes of the book and may be useful to groups of health care professionals when they study it. The questions are keyed to the chapters of the book.

Preface

1. What is the aim of this book?

2. What is an error? What is harm? What is a system? What are the possible relationships among and between them?

3. Systems designed to produce something are never designed to be "safe" first. They are designed first to produce what they are supposed to produce. It is hoped that they will also be safe at an acceptable level. The safety of the system usually relies on a series of protective methods and actions. The functioning of these protective methods is assumed, but often not known directly by the operator of the system. The limit of their safety may or may not be known by the operator. Most of the advanced systems of medical care are hazardous (i.e., they have the capacity to induce substantial harm). Workers are often engaged in trying to mitigate the potential for harm in these systems. What is the responsibility of "responsible medical professionals" to know the empiric limits of safety of the system? Is an "error" different when the harm arises from a known, predictable risk from when the "error" arises from an unexpected circumstance or unrecognized risk? What responsibility do medical providers have for trying to mitigate errors and harm? What actions or activities can they engage in to increase the safety of the system?

Chapter 1. Narrative Ethics

1. Following medical harm, how might a provider's lack of disclosure be construed as a "lack of compassion"?

2. How is the patient's "story, voice, and perspective" important in the context of clinical care? How does the patient's story help clinicians develop what Hilfiker describes as "an ethical framework in which to work"? How does the patient's narrative compare and contrast with the "clinical account"?

3. Does the use of the provider's personal narrative condition the accounts of medical care-induced harm? How? Does a narrative about "who" is responsible diminish the contribution that the context or system might play? How might a "narrative" convey the contribution that the context and system might have made in the production of harm?

4. How is the "view from below" (the one harmed) different from the "view from the side" (a person trying to understand what failed)? Do both views contribute to forgiveness?

Chapter 2. Physicians' Narratives

1. What types of stories can physicians tell after a patient has been harmed? How can physicians' stories be used to inform medical education? How can they be used to affect patient care?

2. How does medical error interfere with the ordinary work of a physician — acknowledging the patient's pain, listening to the patient's voice, and responding to the patient's needs?

3. How does disclosure support and build the patient-physician relationship?

4. Sidney Dekker, author of *The Field Guide to Human Error Investigations*, invites us to consider the difference between explaining system failure and excusing it. He suggests the value of "re-situating" oneself into the situation facing a person as the system failure is created, trying carefully to avoid the problem of hindsight bias — which makes understanding so difficult. Creating a story that helps explain the failure can help us learn about the processes that have been involved in producing the harm. How can such a story complement the narrative accounts of Hilfiker, Gawande, and Ofri?

5. While often referred to, the "hidden curriculum" can also be thought of as another example of the "experiential learning" described by David Kolb (fig. A.1). Where do the teacher's and the learner's values inform the learner's experiential learning? Compare and contrast the effect of observed behaviors and espoused values on what is learned.

Chapter 3. Patients' and Families' Narratives

1. What is the "understanding" that patients want after health care–induced harm? What might be included in narrative accounts that might foster appreciation and understanding of the "view from below"?

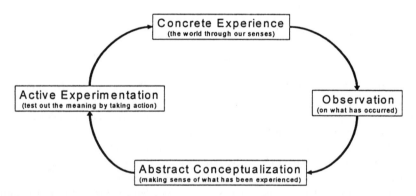

Fig. A.1. Experiential learning model. Adapted from David Kolb (1984).

2. How can patient and family narratives be used to inform patient care and medical education?

3. Is disclosure of medical harm an individual or a system responsibility? or both? How can individuals meet their personal responsibility to disclose while maintaining their responsibility to the system?

4. Is there empirical evidence of "what patients want" and about alternative methods of meeting those needs? What are the possible constraints that are operating and that may condition the methods for providing patients with what they want? How might those constraints serve as barriers to giving patients what they want? How could the effects of these barriers or constraints be mitigated?

Chapter 4. Disclosure

1. In what ways is Bonhoeffer's insistence on framing truth telling as a practice embedded in human relationships and social contexts useful in health care–caused harm? How might Bonhoeffer's essay on "speaking the truth" be used in medical education? How do his principles relate to the patient-physician relationship?

2. How does telling the truth about unintended medical harm compare and contrast with Bonhoeffer's dilemma about telling the truth to Judge Manfred Roeder?

3. How does telling the truth about medical error honor Bonhoeffer's "view from below"?

4. What alternative "authorities" are operating for physicians — in addition to the hospital?

5. Why might some physicians not be able to admit that they are capable of making errors? Why is that? Why is that? Why is that? Why is that?

Chapter 5. Apology

1. How might state "I'm sorry" laws affect the patient-physician relationship in the aftermath of medical harm? What are the benefits and limitations of these laws?

2. How is apology a necessary but insufficient act in the aftermath of medical harm?

3. When the physician contributed to the system failure that resulted in harm to the patient, what should he or she say?

Chapter 6. Repentance

1. How does fair compensation after medical harm relate to the core principles of the patient-physician relationship? Minow asserts that reparations may satisfy the injured party's need for apology (but not vice versa). What is the basis for this assertion?

2. When medical injury occurs in the absence of negligence, how is the idea of individual provider responsibility counterintuitive from a system perspective? How might the concept of individual responsibility promote or deter a system's approach to harm, and to prevention of future harm?

3. How do the compensation systems of Lexington VAMC, CHW, and COPIC compare and contrast with compensation gained through civil litigation and the tort system? What might prevent more widespread adoption of the Lexington Model in the United States?

4. How is repentance necessary but insufficient for forgiveness?

5. If we established a fee-for-time reimbursement basis for lawyers, what process changes might be necessary to "make it worth their time" to help secure compensation for "harmed" patients?

Chapter 7. Forgiveness

1. What is "cheap grace"? How does cheap grace subvert the relational character of forgiveness? What is omitted when cheap grace supplants the relational process?

2. Compare and contrast Jewish and Christian traditions of forgiveness. How is the human agency particularly important in the Jewish tradition? How does the Christian tradition emphasize one's relationship with God over the human relationship? How might this Christian tradition omit the human relational aspect of forgiveness? Why is it necessary to recognize that Christian and Jewish traditions of forgiveness are characteristic of Western norms and culture? How might this recognition inform expectations for members of other cultures?

3. If Hindu and Buddhist traditions — traditions in which the concept of self is not normatively independent from other persons — offer an alternative frame when considering harm that may have been produced by a system, what would be the advantages and disadvantages of constructing a model based on this tradition? What might such a model be? Similarly, if there isn't an exact construct of forgiveness in such traditions, but rather "compassion" or "suffering with," what might a blended construct of "forgiveness-compassion" be like?

4. How does the " 'hair-shirt' ritual" as practiced in surgical morbidity and mortality (M&M) conferences involve surgeons in the ritual of forgiveness? How does it fail to meet obligations to injured patients? How does it fail to bring "self-forgiveness" to involved clinicians? Are these rituals conducted in an environment of system literacy or illiteracy? What is the significance of the latter? What might be done to change M&M conferences so that they foster understanding of the actual mechanisms of harm?

5. Does "missing the mark" include methods for "setting the mark" or identifying the mark? predicting the mark? making the mark? Missing the mark has been described as a technical error, a risk management problem, a moral wrong, an injustice, a sin, and an example of spiritual and psychological devastation. Why these? Are there other ways of framing "missing the mark?" Do these different ways complement one another in finding the whole truth?

6. Is an honest and forthright risk management policy that puts patients' interests first a "priority" or a "precondition" for transparent, truthful health care work?

Chapter 8. Ethical Action

1. What are the many kinds of medical mistakes? Does forgiveness proceed similarly for all types?

2. Berlinger calls for providers to be "personally accountable even in cases of systems error." She notes that some patients and families may resist explanations that "do not adequately hold individual responsibility for actions that could have been set in motion only by these individuals." In contrast, Dekker portrays the hazards inherent to

systems and notes that people within systems actually prevent many system errors by their diligence and individual actions.

3. What are the roles of "personal accountability" and system accountability? How do individuals involved at the point of medical harm share responsibility with the system? When might pressure for "individual action" obscure system design failure? What role should individuals and systems play in the trilogy of disclosure, apology, and repentance?

4. What might individuals and groups within a health care setting do to help lessen the personal emotional impact that caregivers experience when they are involved in care that results in inadvertent medical harm? How might sense-making (understanding the context, the sequence of events, and the observations and logic of operators) help both the individual and the system deal with these emotions? How might sense-making help to reduce medical harm to future patients?

5. What tactics might health care providers, particularly physicians, use to take advantage of their power and position and avoid or minimize admission of error? How might awareness of patients' vulnerability and the "view from below" help providers to avoid these tactics?

6. What spiritual, mental health, and medical care can be offered when appropriate to allow patients and families to heal from medical harm? If you were responsible for the curriculum, what might hospital chaplains need to know about the production of health care–caused harm?

7. Does the concept of organizational truth telling include truth about organizational capability, design, and analysis?

Notes

Preface

1. The report was published as Kohn, Corrigan, and Donaldson 2000. Even according to *conservative* estimates of the number of deaths resulting from medical error (44,000), "More people die in a given year as the result of medical errors than from motor vehicle accidents (43,458), breast cancer (42,297), or AIDS (16,516)." The "national costs" of harmful medical mistakes—the combined costs of health care, lost income, and other expenses resulting from these injuries—"are estimated to be between $17 billion and $29 billion, of which health care costs represent over one-half." Ibid., 1–2.

2. "The veil of ignorance" is described in Rawls 1971, 136–42. For an overview of "strong objectivity" and other feminist standpoint epistemologies, see Harding 1991. For Foucault's theory of "disqualified knowledges," see Foucault and Gordon 1980, 81–85. For a comparative reading of Bonhoeffer and Levinas on the "Other," see Bongma 1997.

3. The classic text on human error is Reason 1990. For an essential discussion of all types of medical harm, including nosocomial infection and harms resulting from inappropriate care, see Sharpe and Faden 1998. Rubin and Zoloth 2000 includes many useful and important essays, notably Lucian L. Leape's authoritative yet concise overview, "Error in Medicine," and also addresses the issue of mistakes made within the context of clinical ethics consultations.

4. Leape, "Error in Medicine," in Rubin and Zoloth 2000, 100, 101.

ONE: Narrative Ethics

1. For a summary and discussion of the disclosure obligation, see chapter 6.

2. Gallagher et al. 2003, 1001.

3. "Medical Errors and Ethics: A Call for Candor without Fear," amednews.com, July 21, 2003: Editorial. Available online at: *www.ama-assn.org/sci-pubs/amnews/amn_03/edsa0721.htm* (accessed July 28, 2003).

4. For an especially helpful description of Kleinman's "explanatory model," see Fadiman 1997, 260–61.

5. Frank 2002, 20–21.

6. Charon and Montello 2002a, ix.

7. Beauchamp and Childress 2001. The phrase "Georgetown Mantra" refers to Georgetown University's influential Kennedy Institute for Ethics, where Beauchamp teaches.

8. Childress, "Narrative(s) versus Norm(s): A Misplaced Debate in Bioethics," in Nelson 1997, 252–71.

9. Ibid., 262.

10. Ibid., 260–64. Childress's critique of narrative overcorrection focuses on interpretations of the "Dax" case, the personal narrative of a severely burned patient that is perhaps the most well-known case study in bioethics.

11. Davis, "It Ain't Necessarily So: Clinicians, Bioethics, and Religious Studies," in Davis and Zoloth 1999, 13–17. The Navajo example comes from Childress 1997, 262.

12. Nelson 1997, xii.

13. Medical humanities scholars such as Tod Chambers also apply literary theory to the case study, a time-honored teaching tool in bioethics. Chambers argues that these "factual" third-person accounts of medical cases are shaped by multiple genre conventions and should properly be read as fiction. Chambers 1999.

14. Hawkins 1993, xi–xii, 1–3.

15. Ibid., 3.

16. Ibid., xi.

17. Ibid., xi. Hawkins identifies a "problem" with Kleinman's model in that it encourages clinicians to view the patient's account not as a coherent narrative from which the physician can learn, but as raw data that the physician must organize into a proper story so that he can then say what it means: "The patient, then, only 'speaks' through the physician's capacity to listen, understand, and interpret" (179n5).

18. Ibid., xii.

19. See Nussbaum 1995.

20. These distinctions were made by Professor La Capra 2003.

21. This not to say that a story an author believes to be an accurate representation of the memory of her own lived experience cannot be factually untrue, in the sense of being a fantasy.

22. "Narrative form alters experience, giving it a definite shape, organizing events into a beginning, a middle, and an end, and adding drama — heightening feelings and seeing the individuals involved as characters in a therapeutic plot. Writing about an experience — any experience — invariably changes it." Hawkins 1993, 14–15.

23. Ibid., xii. Concerning the difference between their goals, Frank writes, "For Hawkins, the 'study of pathography' has as its goal 'in restoring the patient's voice to the medical enterprise' . . . my goal is restoring the patient's voice to the patients themselves, or enhancing a developing self-consciousness among ill people that they are more than medical patients." Frank 1997, 31–49, at 48n15.

24. Hawkins 1993, 160.

25. Ibid., 161.

26. Consider, for example, one of the greatest examples of the form, Dorothy Sayers's *The Nine Tailors*, in which a suspicious death (of a thoroughly unlikeable character, admittedly) is assumed to be and investigated as a crime, then determined to have been a bizarre accident. The detective fiction of Karel Capek, who introduced the genre into Czech literature in the 1920s, and, more recently, of Alexander McCall Smith, in his novels set in Botswana, often have little to do with crime-solving and more to do with investigating puzzling events or probing moral dilemmas. See Capek 1994, vii–xii.

27. For Sacks's description of the etiology of the clinical tale, see Sacks 1990, vii–ix.

28. Bonhoeffer 1997, 17; see also chapter 4, n18.

29. Hilfiker 2001, 255.

30. D. Bonhoeffer, *Ethics*, trans. N. H. Smith (New York: Simon and Schuster/ Touchstone, 1995), 241. For a further discussion of this material, see chapter 4.

31. Albert Wu makes this point when he describes the physician in the aftermath of error as the *second* victim of that error. Wu 2000, 726–27.

T W O : Physicians' Narratives

1. The Harvard Medical Practice Study includes the following publications, which are often referred to, in the following order, as "Harvard study" 1, 2, 3, and so on: Brennan et al. 1991; Leape et al. 1991; Localio et al. 1991; Weiler et al. 1993; Weiler, Newhouse, and Hiatt 1992; and Johnson et al. 1992.

2. Spence 2001, 1934.

3. Bewtra 2002, 22.

4. Di Bisceglie 2002, 1688.

5. See *bmj.bmjjournals.com/advice/sections.shtml#practice*, under "Fillers" (accessed March 25, 2004).

6. Davies 1994.

7. Anonymous 2000.

8. Hilfiker 1984. A slightly revised version of this article appears as a chapter entitled "Mistakes," in Hilfiker 1985, 72–86. All quotations refer to the original article. According to the biographical note in Hilfiker (1985), the author was born in 1945 and so would have been 39 years old when "Facing Our Mistakes" was published, and 33 years old at the time of the incident described at the beginning of this article.

9. In accounts of error that are written by clinicians who practice in the United States, it is sometimes hard to figure out what went wrong or who was responsible. On the one hand, confronting one's own fallibility is one of the conventions of the *Bildungsroman* of medical school or residency, in which early-career physicians recall, in painstaking detail, their technical, professional, and moral indoctrination into the culture of medicine. In an especially popular example of this genre, Perri Klass writes "mistakes are how you learn" (Klass 1987, 94). Yet when Klass herself describes a possible mistake that she (evidently) made, she distances herself from this incident by adopting a narrative device that she uses nowhere else in her book. At the beginning of the chapter that includes the incident, Klass describes the members of a team on duty over a weekend. One of the students on the team "is more than a little like me . . . We can call her Elizabeth, which is, in fact, my middle name" (Klass 1987, 251). It is "Elizabeth" who is directed to inject Dilantin into a patient's IV line; it is "Elizabeth" who may have delivered the drug too quickly, causing the patient's blood pressure to plummet; it is "Elizabeth" "who is trembling from having almost killed someone" (Klass 1987, 267). Klass is not on duty this weekend; it is "Elizabeth's" life and "Elizabeth's" mistake that she is narrating.

10. Anonymous focus group participant, quoted in Gallagher et al. 2003, 1005.

11. Gawande, "When Doctors Make Mistakes," in Gawande 2002, 47–74. All quotations refer to this version of the text.

12. Ofri, "M & M," in Ofri 2003, 188–207. All quotations refer to this version of the text.

13. Pierluissi et al. 2003, 2838.

14. Another chapter in Gawande's book, "When Good Doctors Go Bad," is a study of a physician for whom substandard care has become the norm. Gawande 2002, 88–106.

15. Wordsworth, *The Prelude*, Book Eleventh, quoted in Ofri 2003, 188.

16. Gallagher et al. 2003, 1004.

17. Ibid., 1004.
18. Konner 1988, 97.
19. Ibid., 356.
20. Klass 1987, 115.
21. Calman 2001, 247.
22. Konner 1988, 46; see also Klass 1987, 115.
23. For a description of this model, see Pollack et al. 2003, 205.
24. For a description of this model, see Shapiro 2003.
25. For a description of this model, see *www.narrativemedicine.org/research.html* (accessed March 25, 2004). See also Charon 2001.
26. Hawkins 1993, 12.
27. This phrase was used by Edward Dauer in his presentation at the January 2002 meeting of the *Promoting Patient Safety* project at the Hastings Center (Dauer 2002).

THREE: Patients' and Families' Narratives

1. Gilbert 1997, 21.
2. Levine 2002.
3. Gawande 2002, 59.
4. Localio et al. 1991, 245. The precise figure cited in the study is 1.53 percent.
5. Ibid., 245.
6. Rowe 2002.
7. Goeltz 2000. A version of this story was read into the record of a U.S. Senate hearing on "Patient Safety: Instilling Hospitals with a Culture of Continuous Improvement," June 11, 2003. References to this version of the story are cited as "Testimony of Roxanne J. Goeltz."
8. Goeltz, "Testimony," 2. The "Testimony" version of this narrative says that Mike's parents were called "shortly after 3:00 a.m.," whereas the earlier version says "4:00 a.m." See Goeltz 2000, 4.
9. Goeltz, "Testimony," 2.
10. Ibid., 2.
11. "M & M" in Ofri 2003, 201. The issue of whether to "clean up" after a death or bad outcome, before allowing the family to see the patient, is a complicated one. A hospital chaplain reports that, at one hospital where she had worked, the practice after an emergency-room death had been to clean up the room "totally"—mop up the blood, empty the trash—before bringing the family to see the patient's body. Although this practice was intended to spare the family any further anguish, the hospital changed its practice after hearing comments from family members who observed the tidied-up room and concluded that the staff did not "do" enough to save their loved one. As a result, according to this chaplain, "we stopped being so neat and clean" (Martha Jacobs, personal communication). What this story has in common with Danielle Ofri's story, which has a different clinical context, is that, in each case, the clinicians made an effort to look at the situation from the perspective of the grieving family and acted in the interest of their emotional well-being. By contrast, the clinicians in Roxanne Goeltz's story evidently made no such effort.
12. Goeltz 2000, 5.
13. Goeltz, "Testimony," 3.

14. Ibid., 3.
15. Ibid., 3.
16. Ibid., 4.
17. Ibid., 4.
18. Ibid., 4.
19. Goeltz 2000, 8.
20. A description of Goeltz's work as a patient-safety advocate is posted on the Web site of Consumers Advancing Patient Safety (CAPS), *http://patientsafety.org/aboutUsGoeltz.htm* (accessed March 27, 2004).

21. Other organizations created by injured patients and their families include PULSE (Persons United Limiting Substandards and Errors in Health Care), which collects and circulates "real life stories and experiences" as a means of providing emotional support to injured patients and their families and as teaching tools for patient-safety advocates and the general public. *www.pulseamerica.org* (accessed March 27, 2004). Another organization, Voice4Patients, whose mission is "empowering patients to be their own health care advocates," also collects and shares "stories and suggestions" from injured patients and their families. www.voices4patients.com (accessed March 27, 2004). Other advocacy-oriented Web sites and publications collect and publish "stories" of medical harm that may be based on personal narratives, interviews, or other primary source material, but are to be distinguished from the actual narratives composed by patients or family members themselves. See, for example, the "Stories of Medical Malpractice" posted on the Web site of the Center for Justice and Democracy, an organization that opposes tort reform initiatives that would curtail patients' rights to sue after medical injuries. *www.centerjd.org/stories/index.html* (accessed March 27, 2004). See also Gibson and Singh 2003.

22. For details of McDougal's case, see Stawicki 2003. Available at *http://news.mpr.org/features/2003/04/25_stawickie_paincap/* (accessed March 15, 2004). The advertisements featuring McDougal's story were produced by two advocacy groups, USAction and the Center for Justice and Democracy; a transcript and a video clip of one ad, entitled "Linda's Story," is available on the USAction website. *www.e-guana.net/organizations/org/06Linda-1.pdf* (accessed March 27, 2004).

23. G. Richard Geier, M.D., quoted in Stawicki 2003.
24. On March 8, 2005, a Google search on "medical error" yielded 124,000 hits.
25. *www.nancylim.org* (accessed March 21, 2004). All subsequent citations refer to documents located on or created for this Web site. Because the Web site includes many different documents, some of which are not paginated, each quotation or other reference is cited with its own note rather than via internal citations. The link for all citations is *www.nancylim.org;* the Web site does not generate links to some individual pages. A narrative description of the location of each citation is provided in the accompanying note; in most cases, sections of the Web site and documents within each section are accessed by using the toolbar on the left-hand side of screen.

26. "Overview," available on home page of Web site, *www.nancylim.org* (accessed March 21, 2004).

27. Details of Lim's initial injury are summarized from the "Birth announcement" document, located on the time line section of the Web site. This document was evidently written and distributed many months before Lim's death (accessed March 21, 2004).

28. Detail's of Lim's symptoms prior to her final hospitalization, and the events leading to her death, are summarized from several documents, including "Letter to friends"

("death announcement") located on the time line section of the Web site and various depositions located on the time line and legal documents sections of the Web site (accessed March 21, 2004).

29. "Overview," home page, *www.nancylim.org* (accessed March 21, 2004).

30. This header appears on all pages of the Web site (accessed March 21, 2004).

31. "Overview" (continuation page), home page, *www.nancylim.org* (accessed March 21, 2004).

32. The most recent update is an article dated August 11, 2002; see "News Forum" (tool bar at top of screen), *www.nancylim.org* (accessed March 21, 2004).

33. Barnes was awarded two "wrongful death" settlements on behalf of his son. The documents describing the terms of each settlement are available at *www.nancylim.org* or see "$750,000 first settlement" and "We settle in chambers" links on the time line section (accessed March 21, 2004).

34. Michael Barnes deposition, 244. Available in Legal Documents, *www.nancylim.org* (accessed March 21, 2004).

35. Michael Barnes deposition, 251–52. Available in Legal Documents, *www.nancylim.org* (accessed March 21, 2004).

36. Michael Barnes deposition, 251, 252. Available in Legal Documents, *www.nancylim.org* (accessed March 21, 2004).

37. The photo of Max is slide 26 in the Photo Biography, *www.nancylim.org* (accessed March 21, 2004).

38. Barnes is trained as an economist and, at the time of his deposition, was working for an economics think tank. See Michael Barnes deposition, 180. Available in Legal Documents, *www.nancylim.org* (accessed March 21, 2004).

39. Readers will notice other parallels between the stories told by Gilbert and Barnes: both stories take place in northern California in the early 1990s, and both authors work for the University of California.

40. "National Agenda for Action: Patients and Families in Patient Safety," Patient and Family Advisory Council, National Patient Safety Foundation 2003, 7. Available at *www.npsf.org/download/AgendaFamilies.pdf* (accessed March 25, 2004).

41. National Agenda for Action 2003, 7, 9.

FOUR: Disclosure

1. American Medical Association, Code of Medical Ethics, Ethical Opinions, E-8.12. Issued March 1981; updated June 1994. Available online at *www.ama-assn.org*, via "Policy Finder" function (accessed March 22, 2004). As Sissela Bok has pointed out, until this clause was added, virtually no code of medical ethics—in any culture, at any point in recorded history—required physicians, as a matter of professional ethics, to be honest with their patients. Bok 1978, xiii, xvi; citation refers to 1989 edition.

2. Hamm and Kraman 2001, 20.

3. Ibid., 20.

4. Bok 1982, xv.

5. Hamm and Kraman 2001, 20.

6. Bonhoeffer 1997b, 130.

7. Bethge 2000, 799.

8. Bethge 2000, 813. Based on Bonhoeffer's notes, which were preserved, Bethge dates

the initial drafting of the essay to April–July 1943, when Roeder's interrogations took place, although Bonhoeffer first mentions the essay several months later, when he has resumed work on it. (Bethge 2000, 811, 813; Bonhoeffer 1997b, 130, 158–59, 163–64).

9. Elshtain 2001, 360.

10. Bok [1978] 1989, 282–86; see also 37ff for Bok's discussion of Kant.

11. Elshtain 2001, 361. The Tegel essay has not been included in the *Ethik* volume of *Dietrich Bonhoeffer Werke* (*DBW* 6), the authoritative scholarly edition (the English translation of this revised edition was published by Fortress Press in 2005), nor in the *DBW* edition of the prison letters, *Widerstand und Ergebung* ["Resistance and Submission"], (*DBW* 8). Rather, "Fragment eines Aufsatzes: Was Heisst die Wahrheit sagen?" has been included in a volume entitled *Konspiration und Haft* ["Conspiracy and Imprisonment"]: *1940–45* (*DBW* 16), which has not yet been translated into English.

12. This functional definition of "full disclosure" within the context of medical harm is derived from the policy and practices of the Lexington (Kentucky) Veterans Administration Medical Center (the "Lexington Model"), whose approach to disclosure is discussed in chapter 6.

13. The following discussion of Bonhoeffer's writings on truth telling is indebted to Elshtain's invaluable close reading and analysis in "Bonhoeffer and Modernity" (Elshtain 2001, 360).

14. D. Bonhoeffer 1995b, 241. All subsequent citations to this work appear in the text.

15. Kant, "On a Supposed Right to Lie from Altruistic Motives," in Bok [1978] 1989, 269. Kant's essay, as well as other primary texts on truth telling, is included in an appendix to Bok [1978] 1989.

16. Kant, in Bok 1979, 269.

17. Ibid., 270–71.

18. Bonhoeffer 1997b, 17n2. In a note on the text, Bethge writes that this passage postdates the rest of the essay (he was one of its three recipients) and suggests it may have been written as late as autumn 1943. More recently, the *DBW* editors date it as "ende 1942?" (Bonhoeffer *DBW* 1998, 8, 38). Bethge's suggestion that Bonhoeffer may have written the passage on the "view from below" as late as autumn 1943, when he was revising the essay on truth telling, is tantalizing.

19. Ibid., 17.

20. Bonhoeffer 1995b, 358. Subsequent references to the Tegel essay have not been cited internally because of the textual problem described in n11: Although this text has traditionally been appended to *Ethics*, it is no longer considered to be part of that work, and thus internal references to *Ethics* may be misleading.

21. Ibid., 359.

22. Ibid., 359.

23. Ibid., 359.

24. Ibid., 359.

25. Ibid., 359–60.

26. R. W. Lovin, "The Christian and the Authority of the State: Bonhoeffer's Reluctant Revisions," *Journal of Theology for Southern Africa* 34 (1981): 32–48, at 41.

27. Bonhoeffer 1995a, 67.

28. Bayley 2001, 153–4; see also Hamm and Kraman 2001, 19.

29. The phrase "moral shelter" is used by S. M. Reverby in her essay, "More than Fact and Fiction: Cultural Memory and the Tuskegee Syphilis Study," Reverby 2001, 26,

28n33. Reverby notes that it was contributed by the "first anonymous reader of this paper."

30. "A spoke in the wheel" is the English rendering of a metaphor within "Bonhoeffer's famous analogy for the church's responsibility in his 1933 essay, 'The Church and the Jewish Question.' There Bonhoeffer says that the church's responsibility in the case of a vehicle run amok (i.e., the German state) is not only to bind up the victims fallen under the wheels but to grab the wheels by the spokes in order to stop them." Green 1997, 224. Green notes that this phrase, although used by several English-language Bonhoeffer scholars and translators, perpetuates an "unfortunate ambiguity" with respect to Bonhoeffer's meaning: "In English, a 'spoke' can be either a part of the wheel itself . . . *or* a stake thrust into the wheel to bring it to a halt." The translation should clearly convey the latter definition.

31. Wu et al. 1997, 772–73.

32. Bonhoeffer 1995b, 365.

33. Bethge 2000, 851. With respect to Bonhoeffer's attention to professional ethics, it is worth mentioning that, within the field of bioethics, Bonhoeffer may be identified as a medical ethicist and somewhat anachronistically claimed as a proto-bioethicist. This identification stems from "The Right to Bodily Life" and related material in *Ethics*, in which Bonhoeffer reflects on euthanasia and eugenics. This material, in turn, was informed by his involvement in efforts to help several German doctors uphold their professional obligation to "do no harm" by refusing to comply with the Nazis' euthanasia policies. See Bethge 2000, 688, Bonhoeffer 1995b, 142–85, in particular 159ff; see also Elshtain 2001, 353–54, and Chapman 1999, the latter of which lists Bonhoeffer among the "major Protestant theologians and ethicists" who were "midwives to the birth of bioethics" (224). According to Bethge, Bonhoeffer "spoke with his father," Karl Bonhoeffer, a prominent physician and retired professor of psychiatry and neurology, "about giving [the doctors] authoritative medical documents that they could use as grounds for refusing to hand their patients over" (688). Historian Michael Burleigh, who has researched the Nazi euthanasia program, writes that "[Karl] Bonhoeffer was and remains a controversial figure," particularly among German historians of medicine, in efforts to understand German attitudes towards euthanasia and eugenics prior to as well as during the implementation of the Nazis' policies. Burleigh 1994, 11–12, 118, 293.

34. Bonhoeffer 1997b, 17.

35. Brody, "The Chief of Medicine," in *The Healer's Power* (1992), 1–25. "The Chief of Medicine" was originally published in Brody 1991.

36. Brody 1992, 1.

37. Ibid., 1.

FIVE : Apology

1. In addition to Cohen 2002, other influential treatments of apology under U.S. law and in alternative dispute resolution include Cohen 1999a, 2000a; Minow 1998; Taft 2000; and Schneider 2000. Cohen provides a highly useful bibliography of recent legal scholarship on apology in Cohen 2002, 819n1. The author is grateful to Lee Taft for alerting her to his forthcoming article, "Apology and Medical Mistake: Opportunity or Foil?" *Annals of Health Law* (in press) (L. Taft, personal communication).

2. Cohen, a law professor and economist, is also a scholar of Jewish ethics; Taft, a

longtime plaintiff's lawyer, who now works as a consultant, has been both a student and a dean at Harvard Divinity School.

3. On the Truth and Reconciliation Commission's use of language and practices derived from religion, see Minow 1998, 55, 78. Minow points out that the TRC neither required offenders to apologize as part of the disclosure of their offenses, nor required those harmed by apartheid to forgive the offenders, although she cites professor and human rights activist Andre Du Toit's comment that, under the leadership of Bishop Desmond Tutu, "the influence of religious style and symbolism" on the TRC was significant.

4. On apology after medical error as cultural expectation, see Berlinger and Wu (2005).

5. Cohen 2002, 824n17.

6. Ibid., 825–26.

7. Dating of statutes and descriptions of case law and pending legislation reflects Cohen (2002), except when the status of legislation has changed subsequent to the publication of Cohen's article; in such cases, dates and descriptions reflect the author's own research.

8. *Tex. Civ. Prac. & Rem. Code* § 18.061 (2003); see also *Calif. Code Ann.* § 1160 (2003); *Fla. Stat. Ann.* § 90.4026 (2002); *Wash. Rev. Code* § 5.66.010 (2003); *Tenn. Evid. Rule* 409.1 (2003).

9. *Mass. Laws Ann.* Ch. 233, § 23D (2003).

10. For a detailed discussion of the background of this law, see Taft, 1151, cited in Cohen 2002, 827.

11. *Ill. S.B. 439* (2001); *Iowa S.S.B. 1071* (2001); *R.I. H.B. 6905* (2002), *R.I.* § 1. *Ch. 9–19 L. of Evid.*; *W.Va. S.B. 587* (2001).

12. *Colo. Rev. Stat. Ann.* § 1 Art. 25 tit. 13 (HB. 1232) (2003).

13. *Oreg. H.B. 3361* §§ 1–3 (2003).

14. *Conn. S.B. 577* (2001); *Hawaii S.B.* 1477 (2001).

15. Cohen finds the Connecticut bill "ambiguous" regarding the protection of admissions of fault, although the lack of reference to "sympathy," which is typical of the majority of "I'm sorry" laws, implies that "apology" is inclusive of sympathy plus admission of fault. See Cohen 2002, 831–32.

16. For a discussion of the Hawaii legislation, see Cohen, "Legislating Apology," 832–3.

17. *Deese et al. v. Carroll City County Hospital et al.* 203 Ga. App. 148, 416 S.E.2d 127 (1992).

18. *Robert L. Phinney and Evelyn E. Phinney v. Robert K. Vinson, M.D.* 158 Vt. 646, 605 A.2d 849 (1992); *Joseph and Mary Senesac v. Associates in Obstetrics and Gynecology and Mary Jane Gray, M.D.* 141 Vt. 310, 449 A.2d 900 (1982).

19. The settlement that Nancy Lim's family was offered following her death was based on the substandard care Lim received during a hospitalization for complications resulting from the initial surgical injury.

20. For a discussion of the automotive context of the Massachusetts law, see Taft, 1151, cited in Cohen 2002, 827. Connecticut's proposed legislation notes that the law would apply to "motorists and others." Jonathan Cohen mentions that the legislative debate over California's law included a description of how the law would apply in the case of a driver who, while using a cell phone, collided with another car. See Cohen 2002, 829.

21. Cohen 2002, 845.

22. For a discussion of media coverage of "I'm sorry" laws in several states, see Cohen 2002, 831.

23. Prager 2000.

24. Larry Wobrock, quoted in Duin 2003.

25. Information about COPIC's role in the passage of HB 1232 comes from the following sources: Appleby 2003, 5B; *COPIC Topics* 2003a.

26. Testimony of Mark A. Levine, M.D. Quoted in *COPIC Topics 86* June 2003, 4.

27. *Colo. Rev. Stat. Ann.* § 1 Art. 25 tit. 13 (HB. 1232) (2003).

28. *COPIC Topics 86* June 2003, 4.

29. Lewis 2003.

30. It is worth noting that nurses involved in cases in which error or negligence is alleged tend to be punished more harshly than physicians, and this may affect nurses' willingness to report mistakes they have made or observed. According to a study conducted by the National Patient Safety Foundation to assess the educational needs of physicians and nurses with respect to improving patient safety, nurses reported that although "it is a part of the nursing task and responsibility to report error," nurses, who "are not generally empowered within the hierarchy of medical professionals," may fail to report error because of "the system's punitive procedural processes," as well as "fear and/or humiliation" and, above all, the belief that reporting errors "will not result in actual change." See VanGeest and Cummins 2003.

31. Taft 2000.

32. Cohen 1999a, 1012.

33. Taft 2000, 1142.

34. Cohen1999a, 1060–61, see also 1064.

35. Taft 2000, 1139.

36. Ibid., 1152–53.

37. The classic text on human factors in systems error is J. Reason, *Human Error* (Cambridge and New York: Cambridge University Press, 1990), at 184.

38. Schneider 2000, page 3 of PDF of article.

39. Lucian Leape, quoted in S. Mencimer 2003.

40. Desmond Tutu, quoted in Schneider 2000, 4. See also Shriver 1995, for a variation on this quote — "If you steal my pen and say 'I'm sorry' without returning the pen, your apology means nothing" (224) — and a description of its context.

41. A recent editorial in a leading medical journal makes a similar point concerning apologies after medical mistakes: "While apologies by definition deal with the *intangible* aspects of injury, they do not eliminate the need to address the tangible aspects as well." Frenkel and Liebman 2004, at 482.

42. Bonhoeffer 1995b, 66.

43. King in Wogaman and Strong 1996, 351.

s i x : Repentance

1. Cohen 1999a, 1067–68.

2. Cohen 1999a, 1065–67.

3. LaFree and Rack 1996.

4. T. Grillo 1991; Lerman 1984.

5. Sidney Zimmet, M.D., quoted in Gardner 2004.

6. G. Richard Geier, M.D., quoted in Stawicki 2003.

7. Lucian Leape, quoted in Mencimer 2003.

8. Sharpe 2003, S10.

9. Minow 1998, 117.

10. Minow 1998, 112.

11. Ibid., 112, 117.

12. Tavuchis 1991, 33.

13. Ibid., 33.

14. Minow 1998, 117.

15. The precise relationship between full disclosure and malpractice suits is still being debated, in large part because there are still so few hard data on the cost-effectiveness of full-disclosure policies that are carried out consistently in practice. As a result, hospitals may be tempted to forego full disclosure in practice until it is "proven" to be cost-effective — at *other* hospitals. This, of course, is a catch-22 and it circumvents the ethical obligation to disclose: if hospitals do not consistently disclose mistakes, there will never be sufficient data to demonstrate whether this practice is cost-effective. See Kachalia et al., 2003, 503.

16. For a description of a recent demonstration project conducted in Pennsylvania that studied the use of early, interest-based mediation in disclosure, with attention to compensation, see Liebman and Hyman July-August 2004, 22–32. For a description of a different approach, which uses mediation to resolve formal malpractice claims, see Brown 1998, 432–40.

17. Lamb et al. 2003, 77.

18. The researchers also found that risk managers who expressed the most concern about malpractice litigation were the ones who were the least likely to disclose mistakes. Lamb et al. 2003, 79.

19. This program is described in detail in Kraman and Hamm 1999. See also Hamm and Kraman 2001 and Kraman 2001.

20. The phrase "Lexington Model" is used by Hamm and Kraman 2001, 21. The phrase "humanistic risk management" is used by Kraman and Hamm 1999, 963. Hamm and Kraman's affiliations are described by legal scholar Jonathan R. Cohen in his analysis of the Lexington Model, which includes interviews with Kraman, Hamm, and other Lexington VAMC staff; see Cohen 2000, 1452.

21. The circumstances of the error that gave rise to the Lexington Model are discussed in Kraman 2001, 254.

22. Kraman and Hamm 1999, 964.

23. Kraman and Hamm 1999, 964; Hamm and Kraman 2001, 21–22.

24. At the Lexington VAMC, the chief of staff discloses mistakes on behalf of the institution and individual responsible parties on the basis that "the ethical obligation is institutional," particularly at a teaching hospital staffed largely by residents (Hamm and Kraman 2001, 23). In his critique of this aspect of the Lexington Model, Albert Wu contends that disclosure is "more naturally" the responsibility of the individual physician who has made the error. See Wu 1999, 971.

25. Kraman and Hamm 1999, 964.

26. Lexington's Full Disclosure Handbook is included in Hamm and Kraman 2001, 21–22.

27. Gerlin 1999. Reprinted in Cohen 2000a, 1448.

28. Contrary to the belief of many physicians outside the VA health care system, patients in this system can sue for malpractice, although they cannot sue physicians personally: "despite being immune from personal inclusion as a defendant, [VA] physicians are deposed, may have to testify, suffer damage to their reputations and, if a settlement or judgment is made, can be reported to the National Practitioner Databank (NPDB) and their state licensure boards." Kraman 2001, 254.

29. Kraman and Hamm 1999, 966.

30. Kraman 2001, 256.

31. Hamm and Kraman 2001, 19.

32. Quoted in Gerlin 1999. Reprinted in Cohen 2000a, 1451.

33. Information about CHW's history was provided by Carol Bayley, CHW's Vice President for Ethics and Justice Education, in a presentation entitled "Changing Behavior Based on Core Values: A Project to Address Medical Mistakes in a Large Health System," at a meeting of the *Promoting Patient Safety* project at The Hastings Center, July 12, 2001, and in subsequent conversations with the author.

34. Background information on the evolution of the "Mistakes Project" was provided by Carol Bayley, personal communication.

35. Bayley 2001, 150.

36. Ibid., 151.

37. Ibid., 158. The CHW Philosophy of Mistake Management is included as the appendix to this article.

38. Ibid., 158.

39. Ibid., 153–54.

40. Ibid., 159.

41. Ibid., 154.

42. Berlinger and Wu (2005).

43. C. Bayley, personal communication.

44. Information about COPIC's "3Rs" program comes from the following COPIC articles and publications (*Copic* [later, *COPIC*] *Topics* is the company's newsletter; *Copiscope* is its risk management publication for physicians): "Copic's 3Rs — A Pilot Program to Recognize, Respond to and Resolve Patient Injury," *Copic Topics* 1999; "3Rs Program Showing Proof of Value of Early Communication," *Copiscope* 2001; "A Simple Way to Prevent Patient Anger, Preserve Good Relationships, and Reduce Lawsuits," *COPIC Topics* 2002; "Disclosing Unanticipated Outcomes to Patients," *Copiscope* 2002; "An Update on the 3Rs Program," *Copiscope* 2003; and *COPIC's 3Rs Program* [newsletter for participants] 1 (2004): 1–2. Additional information about the COPIC program comes from Appleby 2003.

45. *Copiscope* 2002, 1.

46. *Copiscope* 2002, 2.

47. *COPIC Topics* 1999, 4.

48. *Copiscope* 2001, 5–6.

49. *Copiscope* 2001, 5; *Copiscope* 2003, 5. According to COPIC risk manager Leslie Taylor, as of December 31, 2003, 1,323 physicians were enrolled in the program (personal communication, March 8, 2004).

50. Richert E. Quinn, VP of Risk Management, Copic Insurance Company, quoted in *COPIC Topics* 1999, 4.

51. *COPIC Topics* 1999, 4.

52. *COPIC Topics* 1999, 5; *Copiscope* 2001, 5; *Copiscope* 2003, 5.

53. *COPIC's 3Rs Program* [participant newsletter], 1.

54. *Copiscope* 2003, 6; *COPIC's 3Rs Program* [participant newsletter], 2; see also Appleby 2003.

55. *Copiscope* 2003, 6; *COPIC's 3Rs Program* [participant newsletter], 2.

56. Kraman 2001, 257.

57. With respect to this trade-off, it is important to remember that the three institutions discussed with respect to their approaches to fair compensation stand in three different relationships to physicians and as a result must structure incentives and obligations differently. COPIC, as an insurer, is able to offer physicians in the 3Rs program unique incentives, such as opportunities to accrue points toward discounted-premium status through consistent enrollment and to earn continuing medical education (CME) credits by completing a seminar on disclosing unanticipated outcomes, but it cannot compel or encourage physicians to participate as a condition of their employment. See *COPIC Topics* 2002, 2; *Copiscope* 2003, 5.

58. Kraman 2001, 256. See also Waters et al. 2003.

59. Kraman 2001, 257.

60. *Copiscope* 2002, 1.

61. *Copiscope* 2002, 2

62. *Copiscope* 2002, 2. COPIC urges physicians to discuss apology scenarios with risk managers before speaking with patients, given that an adverse outcome that does not result from a mistake does not require a fault-admitting apology.

63. Taft 2000, 1152–53.

64. In addition to the national no-fault compensation programs in the three Scandinavian countries and in New Zealand, "[s]everal small medical no-fault schemes have also been implemented in the United States to compensate specific injury types, including the Florida and Virginia schemes for birth-related neurological injury and the National Vaccine Injury Compensation Program." Studdert and Brennan 2001b, 229.

65. Studdert and Brennan 2001a, 219.

66. Studdert and Brennan 2001b, 219, 222.

67. *Copiscope* 2001, 5–6.

68. See Luke 6:31; also Matthew 7:12.

69. *Copiscope* 2002, 3.

70. Quoted in Appleby 2003.

71. Rasmussen 1993, 113.

72. Sharpe 2000, 185.

73. Bayley, "Medical Mistakes and Institutional Culture," in Sharpe 2004, 104.

SEVEN: Forgiveness

1. Kohn, Corrigan, and Donaldson 2000. This citation refers to the published version of the report, which was released in November 1999.

2. Davis, "It Ain't Necessarily So: Clinicians, Bioethics, and Religious Studies," in Davis and Zoloth 1999, 10, 12–17.

3. The eschatological dimension of *kairos* is discussed in Cooper-White 1995, 262.

4. In researching this chapter, the author benefited from many conversations, on Hindu and Buddhist traditions, in particular, with visiting international scholars at The Hastings Center.

5. Kleinman 1995, 13.

6. The "one in five" statistic was cited by Bryan Liang, Professor of Law and Medicine, Southern Illinois School of Law, at the July 12–13, 2001 meeting of the *Promoting Patient Safety* project at The Hastings Center. The "one in four" statistic is derived from data reported by the 2000 U.S. Census (Laing 2001).

7. Werblowsky and Wigoder 1997, s.v. "sin"; Freedman 1992, s.v. "sin, sinners."

8. Ibid.

9. Werblowsky and Wigoder 1997, s.v. "atonement."

10. Werblowsky and Wigoder 1997, s.v. "atonement." *Kapparah* and *Kippur* share the same root.

11. Werblowsky and Wigoder 1997, s.v. "*tiqqun 'olam.*" The author is grateful to Charles L. Bosk for drawing her attention to the recovered tradition of *tikkun 'olam* with respect to the contemporary observance of *Yom Kippur* in particular.

12. Mt 6:12 (New Revised Standard Version).

13. Lk 11:4 (NRSV).

14. Bonhoeffer, "Costly Grace," in Kelly and Godsey 2001, 43.

15. M. Luther, in *Works*, 1958, 223–9. Anthologized in Hodgson and King 1985, 185.

16. Bonhoeffer 2001, 43.

17. Cooper-White 1995, 253, 255.

18. Bonhoeffer 1995b, 87.

19. In addition to sponsoring A Campaign for Forgiveness Research, the Templeton Foundation's Program to Encourage the Scientific Study of Forgiveness has commissioned an annotated bibliography of social science research on forgiveness, which has been included in Worthington 1999. The Web site of A Campaign for Forgiveness Research includes descriptions of the 46 projects fully or partially funded as of 2001. Available online at: *http://forgiving.org* (accessed June 30, 2004).

20. See *www.ukans.edu/7Eforgive/* (accessed December 8, 2001).

21. See *www.stanford.edu/7Ealexsox/forgiveness_article.htm* (accessed December 8, 2001).

22. Clinical studies of forgiveness include Freedman and Enright 1996 and Kaminer et al. 2001. Enright is also the founder and director of the International Forgiveness Institute, www.forgiveness-institute.org (accessed December 12, 2001).

23. Bosk 1979. Subsequent quotations and references are cited internally.

24. See Bosk 1979, 127–46, for additional description and analysis of this ritual.

25. Cross and Livingstone 1997, s.v. "hair-shirt."

26. Hatchett 1980, 449–50.

27. For a discussion of Austin's taxonomy, see Grimes 1996, 285, 288.

28. The author is grateful to the anonymous reviewer of an earlier version of this chapter for this observation.

29. Albert Dreisbach, Department of Internal Medicine, Tulane University School of Medicine, New Orleans, Louisiana, personal communication.

30. Lyla Correoso, attending physician, Calvary Hospital, Bronx, New York, personal communication; staff chaplain, personal communication.

31. A. Dreisbach, personal communication.

32. A. Dreisbach, personal communication.

33. L. Correoso, personal communication; Donna Conroy, student chaplain, Calvary Hospital, Bronx, New York, personal communication. (n.b.: Conroy is also a former nurse.)

34. L. Correoso, personal communication; D. Conroy, personal communication.

35. A. Dreisbach, personal communication; Curtis Hart, Director of Pastoral Care, New York–Presbyterian Hospital and Lecturer, Division of Medical Ethics, Weill-Cornell Medical College, New York, New York, personal communication.

36. C. Hart, personal communication.

37. D. Conroy, personal communication.

38. D. Conroy, personal communication.

39. Kraman and Hamm 1999, 964.

E I G H T : Ethical Action

1. Gawande, "When Doctors Make Mistakes," in Gawande 2002, 57.

2. Anonymous focus group participant, quoted in Gallagher et al. 2003, 1004.

3. See, for example, Wu et al. 1997, 770–75; and Wu 1999, 971.

4. Gallagher et al. 2003, 1004.

5. Gilbert 1997, 37, 72, 337.

6. Levine 2002, 241, 239.

7. Hilfiker, 1984, 121.

8. The author is grateful to Rev. Dean Weber for the observation that the notion of "systems error" or "collective guilt" may be unpalatable in principle to persons or groups who may conceptualize error or sin as actions that can be initiated only by individual moral agents.

9. Norris 1993, 79.

10. Gallagher et al. 2003, 1006.

11. Ibid., 1006.

12. Wu 2000, 726, 727.

13. Pollack et al. 2003, 205.

14. The author is grateful to Jonathan Cohen for his observation concerning one possible legal problem with proposals that might describe hospital chaplains or other clergy as "confessors" for clinicians who have made mistakes. According to Cohen, the "priest-penitent privilege," which protects clergy from being forced to reveal information that has been disclosed to them within the context of a religious "confession" (but not outside of this context), could arguably be invoked in such a way as to detract from the ability of an institution to fully investigate a clinician's role in a mistake (personal communication). Sissela Bok also offers an important critique of institutional practices that ostensibly uphold "confidentiality," but in fact work against the interests of patients and other vulnerable persons by ensuring that key information is kept secret; see Bok 1982, 133–35. As such, although professional chaplains may have the potential to serve as important resources in helping clinicians to address the emotional dimensions of medical mistakes, care should be taken to avoid any misunderstandings concerning the "confessional" nature of these activities. For much the same reason, the term "confessor," with its connotations of secrecy, should perhaps be avoided as a way of characterizing any person or function involved in the resolution of medical mistakes.

15. American Medical Association, Ethical Opinions, E-8.12. Issued March 1981; updated June 1994. Available online at: www.ama-assn.org, via "Policy Finder" function (accessed March 22, 2004).

16. American College of Physicians, Ethics Manual, "Disclosure." Available at: www.acponline.org/ethics/ethicsman.htm. (accessed September 12, 2002).

17. *Comprehensive Accreditation Manual for Hospitals,* LD5–LD5.3. Joint Commission on Accreditation of Healthcare Organizations, 2003.

18. Bok 1982.

19. The author is indebted to Rev. Curtis Hart for his observations concerning the "corrosive" effect on health care providers of withholding the truth about medical mistakes from patients. Personal communication.

20. Goeltz told this story during her presentation at "Improving Patient Safety In Your Institution: Issues and Resources for Hospital Leaders," Connecticut Hospital Association, April 14, 2003.

21. Bayley 2001, 158.

22. Ofri 2003, 189.

23. Fadiman 1997.

24. For Kleinman's critique of the word "noncompliance" as used by physicians, see Fadiman 1997, 261.

25. Quill, Arnold, and Platt 2001, 551–55.

26. Quill, Arnold, and Platt 2001, 554.

27. Gilbert 1997, 218–19.

28. Hamm and Kraman 2001, 23.

29. Hamm and Kraman 2001, 23. At the Lexington VAMC, the chief of staff is responsible for disclosing errors to patients on behalf of the institution.

30. For a summary of these critiques, see chapter 6, n24.

31. Berlinger and Wu (2005).

32. Hamm and Kraman 2001, 24.

33. The author is indebted to Rev. Curtis Hart for his observations on these issues. Personal communication.

34. Donna Conroy, personal communication.

35. Donna Conroy, personal communication.

36. See Wu 1999, 971.

37. A curriculum on death and dying, developed by professional chaplains for medical students, describes the following scenarios in which a chaplain should be in the room when a clinician is breaking bad news to a patient: "[a] patient is going to be given a difficult or terminal diagnosis . . . especially when there is no family present"; "[a] patient's prognosis is going to be changed from curable [,] or in remission, to terminal." Spencer 2000, 27. Quoted with permission.

38. This question has arisen in several states concerning the privacy of the counseling records of survivors of rape or sexual abuse, most notably with respect to the Roman Catholic Church's sexual abuse crisis. In 2002, the Roman Catholic bishops pledged to provide "counseling" to survivors of sexual abuse by priests. In some dioceses, survivors and even counselors were not informed that defense attorneys might subpoena counseling records. In other dioceses, counseling was used as a pretext for obtaining information from survivors, or for persuading them not to sue.

39. Dauer, Marcus, and Thomasson 1999, 10.

40. Grillo 1991, 1545–1610. Citation refers to LexisNexis version of this article: 1–62, at 22–3.

41. Grillo also points out that transference and countertransference occur in doctor-patient relationships; see n225.

42. Cooper-White 1995, 253–57; Fortune 1988, 215.

43. "National Agenda for Action: Patients and Families in Patient Safety," (Patient and Family Advisory Council, National Patient Safety Foundation, 2003), 4. Available online at: www.npsf.org/download/AgendaFamilies.pdf (accessed March 25, 2004).

44. Description of Service of Remembrance provided by Rev. Paul Derrickson, Coordinator of Pastoral Services, Milton S. Hershey Medical Center, Hershey, Pa. Personal communication.

45. Hilfiker, 2001, 255.

References

American College of Physicians. 2002. *Ethics manual: Disclosure.* www.acponline.org/ ethics/ethicman.htm#disclose.

American Medical Association. 1994. *Code of medical ethics.* www.ama-assn.org/ama/pub/ category/8497.html.

Anderlik, M. R., R. D. Pentz, and K. R. Hess. 2000. Revisiting the truth-telling debate: A study of disclosure practices at a major cancer center. *Journal of Clinical Ethics* 11 (3): 251–59.

Andrew, L. B. 2000. Forgiveness essential to healing profession. *American Medical News* September 11, p. 44.

Anonymous. 2000. Looking back. *British Medical Journal* 320 (7237): 812.

Appleby, J. 2003. Insurers, hospitals try apologies for errors. *USA Today*, March 5.

Banja, J. 2001. Moral courage in medicine: Disclosing medical error. *Bioethics Forum* 17 (2): 7–11.

Barach, P., and D. M. Berwick. 2003. Patient safety and the reliability of health care systems. *Archives of Internal Medicine* 138 (12): 997–98.

Bartels, W. K. 2000. The stormy seas of apologies: California evidence code section 1160 provides a safe harbor for apologies made after accidents. *Western State University Law Review* 28:141–57.

Bayley, C. 2001. Turning the Titanic: Changing the way we handle mistakes. *HEC Forum* 13 (2): 148–59.

———. 2004. Medical mistakes and institutional culture. In *Accountability: Patient safety and policy reform*, ed. V. A. Sharpe, 99–117. Washington, D.C.: Georgetown University Press.

Beaglehole, R. 2001. Uses of error: Clinical and epidemiological. *Lancet* 357 (9250): 140.

Beauchamp, T. L., and J. F. Childress. 2001. *Principles of biomedical ethics.* 5th ed. New York: Oxford University Press.

Bedell, S. E., K. Cadenhead, and T. B. Graboys. 2001. The doctor's letter of condolence. *New England Journal of Medicine* 344 (15): 1162–64.

Berlinger, N. 2003a. Avoiding cheap grace: Medical harm, patient safety, and the culture(s) of forgiveness. *Hastings Center Report* 33 (6): 28–36.

———. 2003b. Broken stories: Patients, families, and clinicians after medical error. *Literature and Medicine* 22 (2): 230–40.

———. 2003c. What is meant by telling the truth: Bonhoeffer on the ethics of disclosure. *Studies in Christian Ethics* 16 (2): 80–92.

———. 2004a. Fair compensation without litigation: Addressing patients' financial needs in disclosure. *Journal of Healthcare Risk Management* 24 (1): 7–11.

———. 2004b. Promoting patient safety: Implications for pastoral care. *Journal of Pastoral Care & Counseling* 58 (1–2): 55–61.

Berlinger, N., and A. W. Wu. 2005. Subtracting insult from injury: Addressing cultural expectations in the disclosure of medical error. *Journal of Medical Ethics* 31:106–08.

Berman, S. 2002. Reporting outcomes and other issues in patient safety: An interview with Albert Wu. *Journal on Quality Improvement* 28 (4): 197–204.

Berwick, D. M. 2003. Errors today and errors tomorrow. *New England Journal of Medicine* 348 (25): 2570–72.

Berwick, D. M., and L. L. Leape. 1999. Reducing errors in medicine. *British Medical Journal* 319 (7203): 136–37.

Bethge, E. 2000. *Dietrich Bonhoeffer: A biography*, revd. and ed. V. J. Bannett, trans. E. Mosbacher et al. Minneapolis, Minn.: Fortress Press.

Bewtra, C. 2002. Uses of error: Learning experiences. *Lancet* 35 (9300): 22.

Blendon, R. J., C. M. DesRoches, M. Brodie, J. M. Benson, A. B. Rosen, E. Schneider, et al. 2002. Views of practicing physicians and the public on medical errors. *New England Journal of Medicine* 347 (24): 1933–40.

Bok, S. 1978, 1989. *Lying: Moral choice in public and private life*. New York: Random House/Vintage Books.

———. 1982. *Secrets: On the ethics of concealment and revelation*. New York: Pantheon.

Bongma, E. 1997. The priority of the other: Ethics in Africa: Perspectives from Bonhoeffer and Levinas. In *Bonhoeffer for a new day: Theology in a time of transition*, ed. J. W. de Gruchy. Grand Rapids, Mich.: William B. Eerdmans.

Bonhoeffer, D. 1995. *Ethics*, trans. N. H. Smith and ed. E. Bethge. New York: Simon & Schuster/Touchstone.

———. 1996. *Konspiration und Haft, 1940–1945*, ed. J. Glenthuj, U. Kabitz, and W. Krèotke. Geutersloh: Chr. Kaiser Verlag.

———. 1997. *Letters and papers from prison*. Enlarged ed. Ed. E. Bethge, trans. R. Fuller and F. Clark. New York: Simon & Schuster/Touchstone Books.

———. 1998. *Widerstand und Ergebung Briefe und Aufzeichnungen aus der Haft*, ed. C. Gremmels, E. Bethge, and R. Bethge. Gèutersloh: Chr. Kaiser Verlag.

———. 2001. *Discipleship*, ed. G. B. Kelly and J. D. Godsey and trans. B. Green and R. Krauss. Minneapolis, Minn.: Fortress Press.

Boodman, S. G. 2002. No end to errors. *Washington Post*, December 3.

Bosk, C. L. 1979. *Forgive and remember: Managing medical failure*. Chicago: University of Chicago Press.

Boylan, M. 2003. Creating value-focused patient safety. *Focus on Patient Safety* 6 (1): 3–4.

Brennan, T. A., L. L. Leape, N. M. Laird, L. Hebert, A. R. Localio, A. G. Lawthers, et al. 1991. Incidence of adverse events and negligence in hospitalized patients. Results of the Harvard Medical Practice Study I. *New England Journal of Medicine* 324 (6): 370–76.

British Medical Association. 2002. *Patient safety and clinical risk*, 1–32. Available online at: www.bma.org.uk.

Brody, H. 1991. The chief of medicine. *Hastings Center Report* 21 (4): 17–22.

———. 1992. *The healer's power*. New Haven, Conn.: Yale University Press.

Brown, M. D. 1998. Rush Hospital's medical malpractice mediation program: An ADR success story. *Illinois Bar Journal* August: 432–40.

Buckley, J. M. 2003. 2003 Legislative activity: Big effort yields big results. *COPIC Topics* 86:1–2.

Burleigh, M. 1994. *Death and deliverance: "Euthanasia" in Germany c. 1900–1945.* Cambridge: Cambridge University Press.

Burrell, D., and S. Hauerwas. 1977. From system to story: An alternative pattern for rationality in ethics. In *Knowledge, value and belief,* ed. H. T. Engelhardt and D. Callahan. Hastings-on-Hudson, N.Y.: Hastings Center.

Burstin, H. R., W. G. Johnson, S. R. Lipsitz, and T. A. Brennan. 1993. Do the poor sue more? A case-control study of malpractice claims and socioeconomic status. *JAMA* 270 (14): 1697–1701.

Burton, S. 2003. The biggest mistake of their lives. *New York Times Magazine,* March 13.

Calman, N. S. 2001. No one needs to know. *Health Affairs* 20 (2): 243–49.

Capek, K. 1994. *Tales from two pockets,* ed. N. Comrada. North Haven, Conn.: Catbird Press.

Catholic Healthcare West. 2002. *CHW standards for mission integration,* 1–12. Catholic Healthcare West, San Francisco.

Chambers, T. 1999. *The fiction of bioethics: Cases as literary texts.* New York: Routledge.

Chapman, A. R. 1999. *Unprecedented choices: Religious ethics at the frontiers of genetic science.* Minneapolis, Minn.: Fortress Press.

Charon, R. 2001. The patient-physician relationship. Narrative medicine: A model for empathy, reflection, profession, and trust. *JAMA* 286 (15): 1897–1902.

Charon, R., and M. Montello, eds. 2002a. Memory and anticipation: The practice of narrative ethics. In *Stories matter: The role of narrative in medical ethics,* ed. R. Charon and M. Montello. New York: Routledge.

———. 2002b. *Stories matter: The role of narrative in medical ethics.* New York: Routledge.

Chassin, M. R., and E. C. Becher. 2002. The wrong patient. *Annals of Internal Medicine* 136 (11): 826–33.

Childress, J. F. 1997. Narrative(s) versus norm(s). In *Stories and their limits: Narrative approaches to bioethics,* ed. H. L. Nelson. New York: Routledge.

Coates, T. J. 2002. Uses of error: Compromise. *The Lancet* 360 (9332): 567.

Cohen, J. R. 1999a. Advising clients to apologize. *Southern California Law Review* 72:1009–69.

———. 1999b. Difficult conversations made easier. *Harvard Negotiation Law Review* 4:305.

———. 1999c. Nagging problem: Advising the client who wants to apologize. *Dispute Resolution Magazine* Spring: 19.

———. 2000a. Apology and organizations: Exploring an example from medical practice. *Fordham Urban Law Journal* 27:1447–82.

———. 2000b. Encouraging apology improves lawyering and dispute resolution. *Alternatives to the High Costs of Litigation* 18 (9): 171.

———. 2001. When people are the means: Negotiating with respect. *Georgetown Journal of Legal Ethics* 14:739.

———. 2002. Legislating apology: The pros and cons. *University of Cincinnati Law Review* 70:819–72.

Cooper-White, P. 1995. *The cry of Tamar: Violence against women and the church's response.* Minneapolis, Minn.: Fortress Press.

COPIC Insurance Company. 2002. A simple way to prevent patient anger, preserve good relationships, and reduce lawsuits. *COPIC Topics* 79:1–2.

COPIC Topics. 1999. Copic's 3Rs — A pilot program to recognize, respond to and resolve patient injury. *COPIC Topics* 62:4–5.

———. 2003a. Our tort reform "creed". *COPIC Topics* 86:4.

———. 2003b. Preserving the physician-patient relationship following unanticipated outcomes. *COPIC Topics* 86:4.

Copiscope. 2001. 3Rs program showing proof of value of early communication. *Copiscope* 104:5–6.

———. 2002. Disclosing unanticipated outcomes to patients. *Copiscope* 110:1–3.

———. 2003. An update on the 3Rs program. *Copiscope* 111:5–6.

Corina, I. 2001. A grieving mother's search for answers leads to patient advocacy. *National Patient Safety Foundation Newsletter* 4:6–7.

Cross, F. L., and E. A. Livingstone, eds. 1997. *The Oxford dictionary of the Christian Church.* Oxford: Oxford University Press.

Dajer, A. J. 2001. Physicians and fate. *New York Times*, April 24.

Dauer, E. A. 1997. Adapting mediation to link resolution of medical malpractice. *Law and Contemporary Problems, Medical Malpractice: External Influences and Controls* 60 (2): 185–218.

———. 2002. Mediation as an alternative to malpractice and as a means to quality improvement, presented at Promoting Safety Project meeting, The Hastings Center, January 18, 2002.

———. 2003. A therapeutic jurisprudence perspective on legal responses to medical error. *Journal of Legal Medicine* 24 (1): 37–50.

Dauer, E. A., L. J. Marcus, and S. M. C. Payne. 2000. Prometheus and the litigators. *Journal of Legal Medicine* 21:159–86.

Dauer, E. A., L. J. Marcus, and G. O. Thomasson. 1999. Transformative power: Medical malpractice mediations may help improve patient safety. *Dispute Resolution Magazine* Spring: 9–11.

Davies, G. F. 1994. Anatomy of a complaint. *British Medical Journal* 308 (June 4): 1515.

Davis, D. S., and L. Zoloth. 1999. *Notes from a narrow ridge: Religion and bioethics*, 9–19. Hagerstown, Md.: University Publishing Group.

de Gruchy, J. W. 1997. *Bonhoeffer for a new day. Theology in a time of transition.* Papers presented at the seventh International Bonhoeffer Congress, Cape Town, 1996. Grand Rapids, Mich.: William B. Eerdmans.

———. 1999. *The Cambridge companion to Dietrich Bonhoeffer.* Cambridge companions to religion. Cambridge: Cambridge University Press.

DeNoon, D. 2003. Admit medical errors, doctors urged. my.webmd.com/content/Article/61/67433.htm.

Di Bisceglie, A. M. 2002. An error rationalized is still a mistake. *The Lancet* 360 (9346): 1688.

Downing, L., and R. L. Potter. 2001. Heartland Regional Medical Center makes a "fitting response" to medical mistakes. *Bioethics Forum* 17 (2): 12–18.

Drayer, J. 1999. The culture of secrecy. www.salon.com/health/feature/1999/12/02/meaculpa/print.html.

Duin, S. 2003. A hammer in one hand, a civil suit on the other. *The Oregonian*, May 29.

Dwyer, S. 1999. Reconciliation for realists. *Philosophy and Public Policy Quarterly* 19 (2/3): 18–23.

Dye, C. 2003. Healthcare by numbers. *New Scientist* 177 (2380): 23.

Editorial. 2003. Medical errors and ethics: A call for candor without fear. *American Medical News*, July 21.

Eikelboom, J. 2002. Uses of error: The tip of the iceberg? *The Lancet* 359 (9324): 2194.

Elshtain, J. B. 2001. Bonhoeffer on modernity: Sic et non. *Journal of Religious Ethics* 29 (3): 345–66.

Emmott, D. 2001. Medical errors in surgery. *Bioethics Forum* 17 (2): 26–31.

Enright, R. D., and B. A. Kittle. 2000. Forgiveness in psychology and the law: The meeting of moral development and restorative justice. *Fordham Urban Law Journal* 27 (5): 1621.

Essex, C. 1997. Consultants who changed my practice. *British Medical Journal* 315 (7109): 315.

Fadiman, A. 1997. *The spirit catches you and you fall down: A Hmong child, her American doctors, and the collision of two cultures.* New York: Farrar, Straus and Giroux.

Fonseka, C. 1996. To err was fatal. *British Medical Journal* 313 (7072): 1640–42.

Fortune, M. M. 1988. Forgiveness: The last step. In *Abuse and religion: When praying isn't enough*, ed. A. L. Horton and J. A. Williamson. Lexington, Ky.: DC Health and Company.

Foubister, V. 2000. Broadening the role of forgiveness in medicine. *American Medical News,* August 21. Available online at: www.ama-assn.org/amednews/2000/08/21/prsbo821 .htm.

Foucault, M., and C. Gordon. 1980. *Power/knowledge: Selected interviews and other writings, 1972–1977.* Brighton, Sussex: Harvester Press.

Foxton, M. 2000. An awful mistake. *The Guardian*, August 19.

Frank, A. W. 1997. Enacting illness stories: When, what, and why. In *Stories and their limits: Narrative approaches to bioethics*, ed. H. L. Nelson. New York: Routledge.

———. 2002. "How can they act like that?" Clinicians and patients as characters in each other's stories. *Hastings Center Report* 32 (6): 14–22.

Freedman, D. N. 1992. *The anchor Bible dictionary.* New York: Doubleday.

Freedman, S. R., and R. D. Enright. 1996. Forgiveness as an intervention goal with incest survivors. *Journal of Consulting and Clinical Psychology* 64 (5): 983–92.

Frenkel, D. N., and C. B. Liebman. 2004. Words that heal. *Annals of Internal Medicine* 140 (6): 482–83.

Gallagher, T. H. 2002. Medical errors in the outpatient setting: Ethics in practice. *Journal of Clinical Ethics* 13 (4): 291–300.

Gallagher, T. H., A. D. Waterman, A. G. Ebers, V. J. Fraser, and W. Levinson. 2003. Patients' and physicians' attitudes regarding the disclosure of medical errors. *JAMA* 289 (8): 1001–7.

Gardner, T. 2004. Board rejects report recommending competency tests for doctors. *San Francisco Chronicle*, March 12. Available online at: http://www.sfgate.com/cgibin/ article.cgi?file=/news/archive/2004/03/12/state2030ESTo148.DTL&type=health (accessed March 14, 2004).

Gawande, A. 2002. *Complications: A surgeon's notes on an imperfect science.* New York: Henry Holt and Company/Metropolitan Books.

Gerlin, A. 1999. Accepting responsibility, by policy. *Philadelphia Inquirer,* September 14.

Gibson, R., and J. P. Singh. 2003. *Wall of silence: The untold story of the medical mistakes that kill and injure millions of Americans.* Washington, D.C.: LifeLine Press.

Gilbert, S. M. 1997. *Wrongful death: A memoir.* New York: W. W. Norton.

Gilmore, L. 2001. *The limits of autobiography: Trauma and testimony.* Ithaca, N.Y.: Cornell University Press.

Goeltz, R. 2000. For my brother. *National Patient Safety Foundation Newsletter* 3 (4): 4–8.

———. 2003. Patient safety: The family member's perspective. Paper presented at Improving patient safety in your institution: Issues and resources for hospital leaders. Connecticut Hospital Association Conference, April 13, 2003.

Goeltz, R., and M. J. Hatlie. 2002. Trial and error in my quest to be a partner in my health care: A patient's story. *Critical Care Nursing, Clinics of North America* 14 (4): 391–99.

Goode, E. 2001a. Letting bygones be bygones is often a challenge. *New York Times,* December 11.

———. 2001b. To err may be human; to forgive is good for you. *New York Times,* May 22.

Grandy, D. 2002. Oops, wrong patient: Journal takes on medical mistakes. *New York Times,* June 18.

Gray, R. H. 2001. Uses of error: Epidemiological and clinical. *The Lancet* 358 (9288): 1173.

Green, B. 1997. Recent Bonhoeffer scholarship in Europe and America. *Religious Studies Review* 23 (3): 221–24.

Grillo, T. 1991. The mediation alternative: Process dangers for women. *Yale Law Journal* 100:1545–1610.

Grimes, D. A. 2002. Uses of error: Uncertainty. *The Lancet* 360 (9341): 1242.

Grimes, R. L. 1996. Ritual criticism and infelicitous performances. In *Readings in ritual studies,* ed. R. L. Grimes. Upper Saddle River, N.J.: Prentice Hall.

Halbach, J. L., and L. Sullivan. 2002. *Medical errors and patient safety: A curriculum guide for teaching medical students and family practice residents.* 2:1–102. Valhalla, N.Y.: New York Medical College.

Hamm, G. M., and S. S. Kraman. 2001. New standards, new dilemmas: Reflections on managing medical mistakes. *Bioethics Forum* 17 (2): 19–25.

Harding, S. G. 1991. *Whose science? Whose knowledge? Thinking from women's lives.* Ithaca, N.Y.: Cornell University Press.

Hatchett, M. J. 1981. *Commentary on the American prayer book.* New York: Seabury Press.

Hawkins, A. H. 1992. Restoring the patient's voice: The case of Gilda Radner. *Yale Journal of Biological Medicine* 65 (3): 173–81.

———. 1993. *Reconstructing illness: Studies in pathography.* West Lafayette, Ind.: Purdue University Press.

Hebert, P. C., A. V. Levin, and G. Robertson. 2001. Bioethics for clinicians: Disclosure of medical error. *CMAJ* 164 (4): 509–13.

Hickson, G. B., E. W. Clayton, P. B. Githens, and F. A. Sloan. 1992. Factors that prompted families to file medical malpractice claims following perinatal injuries. *JAMA* 267 (10): 1359–63.

Hickson, G. B., C. F. Federspiel, J. W. Pichert, C. S. Miller, J. Gauld-Jaeger, and P. Bost. 2002. Patient complaints and malpractice risk. *JAMA* 287 (22): 2951–57.

Hilfiker, D. 1984. Facing our mistakes. *New England Journal of Medicine* 310 (2): 118–22.

———. 1985. *Healing the wounds: A physician looks at his work.* New York: Pantheon Books.

———. 2001. From the victim's point of view. *Journal of Medical Humanities* 22 (4): 255–63.

Hobbs, R. 2002. Uses of error: Checks and balances. *The Lancet* 360 (9328): 254.

Hodgson, P. C., and R. H. King, eds. 1985. *Readings in Christian theology.* Minneapolis, Minn.: Fortress Press.

Horwitz, J., and T. A. Brennan. 1995. No-fault compensation for medical injury: A case study. *Health Affairs* 14 (4): 164–79.

Huyucke, L. I., and M. M. Huyucke. 1994. Characteristics of potential plaintiffs in malpractice litigation. *Annals of Internal Medicine* 120 (9): 792–98.

Johnson, C. K. 2003. Patients want information, apology after error. *Spokane Spokesman-Review*, March 13.

Johnson, D. R., S. C. Feldman, H. Lubin, and S. M. Southwick. 1995. The therapeutic use of ritual and ceremony in the treatment of post-traumatic stress disorder. *Journal of Traumatic Stress* 8 (2): 283–98.

Johnson, W. G., T. A. Brennan, J. P. Newhouse, L. L. Leape, A. G. Lawthers, H. H. Hiatt, et al. 1992. The economic consequences of medical injuries: Implications for a no-fault insurance plan. *JAMA* 267 (18): 2487–92.

Joint Commission on Accreditation of Healthcare Organizations. 2003. *Comprehensive accreditation manual for hospitals*. Chicago: Joint Commission Resources.

Kachalia, A., K. G. Shojania, T. P. Hofer, M. Piotrowski, and S. Saint. 2003. Does full disclosure of medical errors affect malpractice liability? The jury is still out. *Joint Commission Journal on Quality and Safety* 29 (10): 503–11.

Kadzielski, M., and C. Martin. 2001. Assessing medical error in health care. *Health Progress* 82 (6): 14–17.

Kaminer, D., D. J. Stein, I. Mbanga, and N. Zungu-Dirwayi. 2001. The Truth and Reconciliation Commission in South Africa: Relation to psychiatric status and forgiveness among survivors of human rights abuses. *British Journal of Psychiatry* 178:373–77.

Keeva, S. 1999. Does law mean never having to say you're sorry? *American Bar Association Journal* 95:64–65.

Kellett, A. J. 1987. Healing angry wounds: The role of apology and mediation in disputes between patients and physicians. *Mississippi Journal of Dispute Resolution* 111:126–27.

King, Jr., M. L. 1996. Letter from Birmingham city jail. In *Readings in Christian ethics: A historical sourcebook*, ed. J. P. Wogaman and D. M. Strong. Louisville, Ky.: Westminster–John Knox Press.

Klass, P. 1987. *A not entirely benign procedure: Four years as a medical student*. New York: Penguin Books/Plume.

Kleinman, A. 1995. *Writing at the margin: Discourse between anthropology and medicine*. Berkeley: University of California Press.

Kluge, E. H. W. 1999. Informed consent in a different key: Physicians' practice profiles and the patient's right to know. *CMAJ* 160 (9): 1321–22.

Kohn, L. T., J. Corrigan, and M. S. Donaldson, eds. 2000. *To err is human: Building a safer health system*. Washington, D.C.: National Academy Press.

Kolb, D. A. 1984. *Experiential learning: Experience as the source of learning and development*. Upper Saddle River, N.J.: Prentice Hall.

Konner, M. 1988. *Becoming a doctor: A journey of initiation in medical school*. New York: Penguin Books.

Kovalchik, M. T. 1991. A piece of my mind: Theo's story. *JAMA* 266 (23): 3340.

Kraman, S. S. 2001. A risk management program based on full disclosure and trust: Does everyone win? *Comprehensive Therapy* 27 (3): 253–57.

Kraman, S. S., L. Cranfill, G. Hamm, and T. Woodard. 2002. Advocacy: The Lexington veterans affairs medical center. *The Joint Commission Journal on Quality Improvement* 28 (12): 646–50.

Kraman, S. S., and G. Hamm. 1999. Risk management: Extreme honesty may be the best policy. *Annals of Internal Medicine* 131 (12): 963–67.

La Capra, D. 2003. Trauma and its after-effects. Presented at *Narrative Medicine: A Colloquium* at Columbia University, May 3, 2003.

LaFree, G., and C. Rack. 1996. The effects of participants' ethnicity and gender on monetary outcomes in mediated and adjudicated civil cases. *Law and Society Review* 30 (4): 767–97.

Lamb, R. M., D. M. Studdert, R. M. Bohmer, D. M. Berwick, and T. A. Brennan. 2003. Hospital disclosure practices: Results of a national survey. *Health Affairs* 22 (2): 73–83.

Landro, L. 2003. Hospitals encourage staff to report medical errors. *Wall Street Journal,* March 25.

Lapetina, E. M., and E. M. Armstrong. 2002. Preventing errors in the outpatient setting: A tale of three states. *Health Affairs* 21 (4): 26–39.

Latif, E. 2001. Apologetic justice: Evaluating apologies tailored toward legal solutions. *Boston University Law Review* 81: 289–318.

Layde, P. M., L. M. Cortes, S. P. Teret, K. J. Brasel, E. M. Kuhn, J. A. Mercy, et al. 2002. Patient safety efforts should focus on medical injuries. *JAMA* 287 (15): 1993–97.

Leape, L., A. M. Epstein, and M. B. Hamel. 2002. A series on patient safety. *New England Journal of Medicine* 347 (16): 1272–74.

Leape, L. L. 2000. Error in medicine. In *Margin of error: The ethics of mistakes in the practice of medicine,* ed. S. B. Rubin and L. Zoloth, 95–111. Hagerstown, Md.: University Publishing Group.

Leape, L. L., T. A. Brennan, N. Laird, A. G. Lawthers, A. R. Localio, B. A. Barnes, et al. 1991. The nature of adverse events in hospitalized patients. Results of the Harvard Medical Practice Study II. *New England Journal of Medicine* 324 (6): 377–84.

Lerman, L. G. 1984. Mediation of wife abuse cases: The adverse impact of informal dispute resolution on women. *Harvard Women's Law Journal* 7:57–113.

Levine, C. 2002. Life but no limb: The aftermath of medical error. *Health Affairs* 21 (4): 237–41.

Lewis, A. 2003. Malpractice measure is "sorry" protection. *Denver Post,* April 13.

Ley, C. 2001. Patient safety: A personal and professional perspective. *National Patient Safety Foundation Newsletter* 4 (2): 6–7.

Liang, B. 2001. Promoting patient safety. Presentation at the *Promoting patient safety* conference at The Hastings Center, July 12, 2001. Available online at: http://fact finder.census.gov (accessed November 18, 2002).

Liebman, C. B., and C. S. Hyman. 2004. A mediation skills model to manage disclosure of errors and adverse events to patients. *Health Affairs* 23 (4): 22–32.

Localio, A. R., A. G. Lawthers, T. A. Brennan, N. M. Laird, L. E. Hebert, L. M. Peterson, et al. 1991. Relation between malpractice claims and adverse events due to negligence. Results of the Harvard Medical Practice Study III. *New England Journal of Medicine* 325 (4): 245–51.

Lowenstein, E., and S. H. Wanzer. 2002. The U.S. Attorney General's intrusion into medical practice. *New England Journal of Medicine* 346 (6): 447–48.

Luther, M. 1958. Against Latomus. In *Luther's Works,* Vol. 32, trans. G. Lindbeck, Philadelphia: Fortress Press. Anthologized in P. C. Hodgson and R. H. King, eds. 1985. *Readings in Christian Theology.* Minneapolis, Minn.: Fortress Press.

Marion, R. 2001. *The intern blues: The timeless classic about the making of a doctor.* New York: Perennial.

Mazor, K. M., S. R. Simon, R. A. Yood, B. C. Martinson, M. J. Gunter, G. W. Reed, et al. 2004. Health plan members' views about disclosure of medical errors. *Annals of Internal Medicine* 140 (6): 409–18.

Meaney, M. 2001. From a culture of blame to a culture of safety: The role of institutional ethics committees. *Bioethics Forum* 17 (2): 32–42.

Mencimer, S. 2003. Casualties of medicine. *Legal Affairs*, May/June 2003. Available online at: www.legalaffairs.org/issues/May-June-2003/story_mencimer_mayjuno3.html (accessed January 6, 2004).

Millenson, M. L. 2003. The silence. *Health Affairs* 22 (2): 103–12.

Miller, F. H. 1986. Medical malpractice litigation: Do the British have a better remedy? *American Journal of Law and Medicine* 11 (4): 433–35.

Minnesota Alliance for Patient Safety. 2002. A call to action: Roles and responsibilities for assuring patient safety, 1–6. Available online at: www.mnpatientsafety.org/pdfs/A%20 Call%20to%20Action.pdf

Minow, M. 1998. *Between vengeance and forgiveness: Facing history after genocide and mass violence.* Boston: Beacon Press.

Molyneux, E. 2001. Uses of error: Lessons learnt. *The Lancet* 358 (9278): 323.

Murphy, D. J. 2002. Uses of error: An obstetric perspective. *The Lancet* 360 (9337): 941.

National Patient Safety Foundation. 2003. Patients and families in patient safety: Nothing about me, without me, 1–12. Available online at: www.npsf.org/download/Agenda Families.pdf.

Nelson, H. L. 1997. *Stories and their limits: Narrative approaches to bioethics.* New York: Routledge.

New York Times. 2002. Errors that kill medical patients, December 18.

———. 2003. The malpractice insurance crisis, January 17.

Norris, K. 1993. *Dakota: A spiritual geography.* New York: Houghton Mifflin.

Nussbaum, M. C. 1995. *Poetic justice: The literary imagination and public life.* Boston: Beacon Press.

Ofri, D. 2003. *Singular intimacies: Becoming a doctor at Bellevue.* Boston: Beacon Press.

Orenstein, A. 1999. Incorporating a feminist analysis into evidence policy where you would least expect it. *Southwestern University Law Review* 28:221–79.

Orlander, J. D., T. W. Barber, and B. G. Fincke. 2002. The morbidity and mortality conference: The delicate nature of learning from error. *Academic Medicine* 77 (10): 1001–6.

Pear, R. 1999. Group asking U.S. for new vigilance in patient safety. *New York Times*, November 20.

Pierluissi, E., M. A. Fischer, A. R. Campbell, and C. S. Landefeld. 2003. Discussion of medical errors in morbidity and mortality conferences. *JAMA* 290 (21): 2838–42.

Pollack, C., C. Bayley, M. Mendiola, and S. McPhee. 2003. Helping clinicians find resolution after a medical error. *Cambridge Quarterly of Healthcare Ethics* 12 (2): 203–7.

Poulter, N. R. 2001. Uses of error: Suppositions and surprises. *The Lancet* 358 (9291): 1448.

Prager, L. O. 2000. New laws let doctors say 'I'm sorry' for medical mistakes. *American Medical News.* Available online at: www.ama.assn.org/amednews/site/bio.htm (accessed November 11, 2003).

Quill, T. E., R. M. Arnold, and F. Platt. 2001. "I wish things were different": Expressing wishes in response to loss, futility, and unrealistic hopes. *Annals of Internal Medicine* 135 (7): 551–55.

Rasmussen, L. 1999. The ethics of responsible action. In *The Cambridge Companion to Dietrich Bonhoeffer,* ed. J. W. de Gruchy. Cambridge: Cambridge University Press.

Rasmussen, L. L. 1993. *Moral fragments and moral community: A proposal for church and society.* Minneapolis, Minn.: Augsburg/Fortress Press.

Rawls, J. 1971. *A theory of justice.* Cambridge, Mass.: Belknap Press of Harvard University Press.

Reason, J. 2000. Human error: Models and management. *British Medical Journal* 320 (7237): 768–70.

Reason, J. T. 1990. *Human error.* Cambridge: Cambridge University Press.

Reitman, V. 2003. Healing sound of a word: 'Sorry'. *Los Angeles Times,* March 24.

Reverby, S. M. 2001. More than fact and fiction. Cultural memory and the Tuskegee syphilis study. *Hastings Center Report* 31 (5): 22–28.

Richards, T. J. 2000. How I almost killed Otis. *Medical Economics* 77 (16): 113–14.

Robinson, A. R., K. B. Hohmann, J. I. Rifkin, D. Topp, C. M. Gilroy, J. A. Pickard, et al. 2002. Physician and public opinions on quality of health care and the problem of medical errors. *Archives of Internal Medicine* 162 (19): 2186–90.

Rosenbaum, M. E., K. J. Ferguson, and J. G. Lobas. 2004. Teaching medical students and residents skills for delivering bad news: A review of strategies. *Academic Medicine* 79 (2): 107–17.

Rothman, E. L. 1999. *White coat: Becoming a doctor at Harvard Medical School.* New York: W. Morrow.

Rothman, M. D. 2003. The error. info.med.yale.edu/intmed/hummed/yihm/regular/mrothman1.htm.

Rowe, M. 2002. The rest is silence. *Health Affairs* 21 (4): 232–36.

Rubin, S. B., and L. Zoloth, eds. 2000. *Margin of error: The ethics of mistakes in the practice of medicine.* Hagerstown, Md.: University Publishing Group.

Ryan, K. 1999. Learning from our mistakes. *British Medical Journal* 318 (7177): 177.

Sacks, O. W. 1990. *The man who mistook his wife for a hat and other clinical tales.* New York: Harper Perennial Library.

Sage, W. M. 1997. Enterprise liability and the emerging managed health care system. *Law and Contemporary Problems, Medical Malpractice: External Influences and Controls* 60:159–210.

Sandercock, P. 2004. Uses of error: A fainting mechanic. *The Lancet* 360 (9329): 305.

Schäfer, S. 2002. A memorable patient: You only see what you know. *British Medical Journal* 326 (583) 583.

Schneider, C. D. 2000. What it means to be sorry: The power of apology in mediation. *Mediation Quarterly* 17 (3). Available online at: www.mediation-matters.com/Resources/apology.htm.

Shapiro, D. 2003. Beyond the blame: A no-fault approach to malpractice. *New York Times,* September 23.

Sharpe, V. A. 2000. Taking responsibility for medical mistakes. In *Margin of error: The ethics of mistakes in the practice of medicine,* ed. S. B. Rubin and L. Zoloth. Hagerstown, Md.: University Publishing Group.

———. 2003. Promoting patient safety: An ethical basis for policy deliberation. *Hastings Center Report Special Supplement* 33 (5): S1–S20.

Sharpe, V. A., and A. I. Faden. 1998. *Medical harm: Historical, conceptual, and ethical dimensions of iatrogenic illness.* Cambridge and New York: Cambridge University Press.

Shriver, D. W. 1995. *An ethic for enemies: Forgiveness in politics.* New York: Oxford University Press.

Shuman, Jr., D. W. 2000. The role of apology in tort law. *Judicature* 83 (4): 180–89.

Shute, N. 2002. Speaking up for patient safety. *U.S. News and World Report*, July 22, 63–66.

Sibbald, B. 2001. Ending the blame game key to overcoming medical error. *CMAJ* 165 (8): 1083.

———. 2002. Reducing medical error: "People doing their best is not enough." *CMAJ* 167 (9): 1047.

Singer, P. A. 2001. Commentary: Learning to love mistakes. *British Medical Journal* 322 (7296): 1238.

Smith, M. L., and H. P. Foster. 2000. Morally managing medical mistakes. *Cambridge Quarterly of Healthcare Ethics* 9 (1): 38–53.

Spence, D. 2001. Uses of error: Knowledge gaps. *Lancet* 358 (9297): 1934.

Spencer, S. 2000. *Patient, physician, and society II: Death and dying faculty guide*. St. Louis: Office of Curricular Affairs, St. Louis University School of Medicine.

Stawicki, E. 2003. Capping the cost of pain and suffering. Minnesota Public Radio, May 16, 2003. Available online at: http://news.minnesota.publicradio.org/features/2003/04/25_stawickie_paincap/ (accessed March 15, 2004).

Studdert, D. M., and T. A. Brennan. 2001a. No-fault compensation for medical injuries: The prospect for error prevention. *JAMA* 286 (2): 217–23.

Studdert, D. M., and T. A. Brennan. 2001b. Toward a workable model of "no-fault" compensation for medical injury in the United States. *American Journal of Law and Medicine* 27 (2–3): 225–52.

Studdert, D. M., E. J. Thomas, B. I. W. Zbar, J. P. Newhouse, P. C. Weiler, J. Bayuk, et al. 1997. Can the United States afford a "no-fault" system of compensation for medical injury? *Law and Contemporary Problems, Medical Malpractice: External Influences and Controls* 60 (2): 1–34.

Swales, J. 2002. Uses of error: The dangers of conformity. *The Lancet* 359 (9321): 1936.

Taft, L. 2000. Apology subverted: The commodification of apology. *Yale Law Journal* 109 (5): 1135–60.

Tanne, J. H. 2002. U.S. doctors and public disagree over mandatory reporting of errors. *British Medical Journal* 325:1055.

Tavuchis, N. 1991. *Mea culpa: A sociology of apology and reconciliation*. Stanford, Calif.: Stanford University Press.

Tieman, J. 2001. Enforcing a new openness: JCAHO to hospitals: Let patients know when their care hasn't met standards. *Modern Healthcare*, June 25. Available online at: www.modernhealthcare.com/search.cms.

VanGeest, J. B., and D. S. Cummins. 2003. An educational needs assessment for improving patient safety: Results of a national study of physicians and nurses. *National Patient Safety Foundation.* 3:1–28.

Veltman, L. 1997. Managing bad results. *Group Practice Journal* 46:26–32.

———. 2001. Should I apologize? A guide for physicians and risk-managers. Presentation at the ASHRM Annual Meeting, October 30.

Verheugt, F. W. A. 2002. Uses of error: Who is to blame? *The Lancet* 360 (9335): 789.

Vincent, C., M. Young, and A. Phillips. 1994. Why do people sue doctors? A study of patients and relatives taking legal action. *The Lancet* 343 (8913): 1609–13.

Volpp, K. G., and D. Grande. 2003. Residents' suggestions for reducing errors in teaching hospitals. *New England Journal of Medicine* 348 (9): 851–55.

Wachter, R. M., K. G. Shojania, S. Saint, A. J. Markowitz, and M. Smith. 2002. Learning from our mistakes: Quality grand rounds, a new case-based series on medical errors and patient safety. *Annals of Internal Medicine* 136 (11): 850–52.

Waters, T. M., D. M. Studdert, T. A. Brennan, E. J. Thomas, O. Almagor, M. Mancewicz, et al. 2003. Impact of the National Practitioner Data Bank on resolution of malpractice claims. *Inquiry* 40 (3): 283–94.

Weeks, W. B., and A. E. Wallace. 2003. Broadening the business case for patient safety. *Archives of Internal Medicine* 163 (9): 1112.

Weiler, P. C., J. P. Newhouse, and H. H. Hiatt. 1992. Proposal for medical liability reform. *JAMA* 267 (17): 2355–58.

Weiler, P. C., H. H. Hiatt, J. P. Newhouse, W. G. Johnson, T. A. Brennan, and L. L. Leape. 1993. *A measure of malpractice: Medical injury, malpractice litigation, and patient compensation*. Cambridge, Mass.: Harvard University Press.

Weiss, R. 1999. Medical errors blamed for many deaths; As many as 98,000 a year in U.S. linked to mistakes. *Washington Post*, November 30.

Wells, J. 2000. Hospitals must disclose doctor errors: Oversight panel seeks to cut preventable patient injuries. *San Francisco Chronicle*, December 24.

Werblowsky, R. J. Z., and G. Wigoder. 1997. *The Oxford dictionary of the Jewish religion*. New York: Oxford University Press.

Wilcox, M. H. 2001. Uses of error: Microbial perils. *The Lancet* 358 (9277): 237.

Willmer, H. 1999. Costly discipleship. In *The Cambridge Companion to Dietrich Bonhoeffer*, ed. J. W. de Gruchy. Cambridge: Cambridge University Press.

Wilson, T., M. Pringle, and A. Sheikh. 2001. Promoting patient safety in primary care. *British Medical Journal* 323 (7313): 583–84.

Witman, A. B., D. M. Park, and S. B. Hardin. 1996. How do patients want physicians to handle mistakes? A survey of internal medicine patients in an academic setting. *Archives of Internal Medicine* 156 (22): 2565–69.

Wogaman, J. P., and D. M. Strong. 1996. *Readings in Christian ethics*. Louisville, Ky.: Westminster John Knox Press.

Worthington Jr., E. L. 1999. *Dimensions of forgiveness: Psychological research and theological perspectives*. Radnor, Pa.: Templeton Foundation Press.

———. 2000. Is there a place for forgiveness in the justice system? *Fordham Urban Law Journal* 27 (5): 1721.

Wu, A. W. 1999. Handling hospital errors: Is disclosure the best defense? *Annals of Internal Medicine* 131 (12): 970–72.

———. 2000. Medical error: The second victim. *British Medical Journal* 320 (7237): 726–27.

———. 2001. Commentary: Doctors are obliged to be honest with their patients. *British Medical Journal* 322 (7296): 1238–39.

Wu, A. W., T. A. Cavanaugh, S. J. McPhee, B. Lo, and G. P. Micco. 1997. To tell the truth: Ethical and practical issues in disclosing medical mistakes to patients. *Journal of General Internal Medicine* 12 (12): 770–75.

Zimmerman, R. 2004. Doctors' new tool to fight lawsuits: Saying "I'm sorry." *Wall Street Journal*, May 18.

Index

fallibility, 14, 25

fair compensation, for medical harm: xiv, 65, 68–69; acceptance of, and waiver of right to sue, 70; and access to mental health services, 107–109; as alternative to litigation, 109; cost-effectiveness of, 70, 74; effects of closed system on, 68, 71; and likelihood of litigation, 67–68, 70; and malpractice insurance, 72–73; moral importance of, 61; payment vs. settlement, implications for physicians, 75–76; programs of, 69–78, 105–106, 131n6; as reparation, 66–67; and repentance, 61, 66; scope of, 75, 109; similarities to no-fault compensation, 77–78; and systems accountability, 66. *See also* no-fault compensation

Forgive and Remember. See Bosk, Charles. L.

forgiveness, x, 9, 14, 81–91; affirming changed behavior, 83; cliches of, ix–x; conditions for, 111; contradictory meanings of, 82–83; and "culture of safety," 81; and detachment, 82–83, 87, 113; ethics of, xi–xii, xv, 92–113; inappropriateness of requesting, 110–111; in Jewish, Christian social ethics, 84–87; and *kairos*, 91; and medical mistakes, xiv–xv, 34; not universal concept, 83; physician expectations for, 90; and principle of justice, 82; as process, 86; and protection of those who cause harm, 86; and relationship, 81, 82, 83; rituals of, 87–91, 110; and salvation, in Christian tradition, 85–86; studies of, xv, 87, 134n19. *See also* Bonhoeffer; *kairos*

Frank, Arthur, 3, 6, 7

"From the Victim's Point of View." *See* Hilfiker, David

Gawande, Atul, 16–20, 22, 23, 24, 26, 30, 93, 94, 107

Gilbert, Elliot, 29–30, 37

Gilbert, Sandra, 29, 31, 37, 39, 95, 104; *Wrongful Death*, 39–30, 104–105

Goeltz, Mike, 32–33, 38

Goeltz, Roxanne, 32–33, 34, 35, 38, 101

Golden Rule, the, 78

guilt, 13, 16, 96; vs. shame, 106–107

"hair-shirt ritual," Morbidity & Mortality Conference as, 88. *See also* Morbidity & Mortality Conference (M&M)

Hamm, Ginny M., 69, 70, 91, 105

harm: intentional vs. unintentional, 7, 8; resolution of, rituals associated with, 8. *See also* medical mistakes

Harvard Medical Practice Study, 11, 19, 31

Hawkins, Anne Hunsaker, 5, 6

health care institution: characteristics of, as small community, 97; role as caregiver, 69, 79; relationship with patient, 37–38

Heartland Forgiveness Project (University of Kansas), 87

Herlan, Raphael, 19–22, 32–33

het' (Hebr.), "miss the mark," usages of, 84

hidden curriculum, 24, 25, 26, 41

Hilfiker, David, 23, 26, 96,113; "Facing Our Mistakes," 14–16; "From the Victim's Point of View," 9–10. *See also* clinical tales

human factors research, 19, 59

"I'm sorry" laws: and admission of fault, 51,52–58, 62; and case law, 54, 129nn17–18; effect on physician practice, 60–61; as legal and policy trend, 52–58, 62; media coverage of, 55–56, 57–58; and physician-patient relationship, 55; as remedy, 60, 61–62; scope of, and medical specialty, 55; states enacted in, 53, 55; states proposed in, 53, 54; Colorado (HB 1232), 53, 55, 56–58; Oregon (HB 3361), 53, 55–56; weaknesses of, 60–61 *See also* fair compensation, programs of

infelicitous performance, concept of, 88–89

injured patients, stereotypes of, 35, 38–39

instant forgiveness, ethics of, 86, 110

Institute of Medicine (IOM), ix, 11, 34, 81

integrity, 4

interrogation, ethics of, 46

Jackson, Shirley, "The Lottery," 97–98

jargon. *See* vocabulary of error

Joint Commission on the Accreditation of Healthcare Organizations, disclosure requirement of, 99–100

justice, 4, 43, 48, 66, 71, 72, 85, 86

Nancy Berlinger is deputy director and associate for religious studies at The Hastings Center in Garrison, New York. She is a graduate of Smith College and holds
the Ph.D. in English Literature from the University of Glasgow and the M.Div. in
Christian Ethics from Union Theological Seminary.